Table of Contents

Introduction

A light southwesterly breeze danced across my face as I stood on the sandy dune, bringing warm air up from the Gulf hundreds of miles away. The smell, the taste, the feel of this breeze brought me back summer after summer for more than thirty years. I watched as some pre–teen boys and girls stood on the sand bar waiting for the next wave to carry them into the shore on their boogie boards. Was the sand bar closer than I remembered it? Had erosion slowly eaten away at the beach, shifting the sands that served as the foundation for the Outer Banks? Or had my life, my worries, minimized the length of nature's ride, of the purity of those few seconds?

I looked south, down the beach directly into the breeze and there he was, just a speck in the distance riding the wind looking for food. It was Billy Pelican, another reason I returned here year after year. In truth, it was just the next in a series of pelicans that flew up and down this beach, every beach on the coast. As a kid, the first time I saw one ride the air currents, ride the waves, I was fascinated and named them all Billy. And like a good friend, they were always here for me.

Someone once gave me an embroidered pillow that read something like "My goal in life is to become the person my dog thinks I am." Maybe that's true, but my dream as a child was to feel like Billy Pelican, to find, to create, those moments where work and play merged into indistinguishable pursuits and pleasures.

When I was twelve or thirteen, I wondered how pelicans learned to surf in this unique way, how something so ugly at rest could be so beautiful in flight. Standing there in that moment, I tried to remember when I lost that sense of wonder. I wondered why it was so easy to obsess over our own ugliness instead of seeking out the beauty of the wind or the rhythm of the waves. Why did so many of us find safety in standing still. Surely, there was a human equivalent to Billy's beauty in flight.

I smiled as Billy skimmed the curl of a wave, his wings tilted slightly toward me, showing me his grayish back. He moved with the subtleties he felt in the wind. My smile remained as he moved farther North and out of sight. I knew this feeling here and now in my thirty-eighth year.

Charles Lindbergh once said, "Building an airplane is easier than the evolutionary process of the flight of a bird. I'd rather be around birds." I had spent the last fifteen years trying to understand my own evolutionary process. I had spent the last ten years teaching others what I learned while applying it to my own life. It seemed so simple now, and yet still so difficult to capture and hold onto.

The water greeted me with its mid-seventies temperature as I dove in and swam out to the sand bar. The current was strong for such a calm day, but my foot finally hit the hard sand. I stood up and walked until the calm water lapped at my waist and the waves rose six inches above my head.

As a squadron of pelicans flew along the waves towards me, the words just came to me—The Most Important Lesson No One Ever Taught Me. That was what I had spent these years learning. It was a lesson no one *could* teach me. They could guide me, but I had to learn it. I had to experience my life, myself. I had to learn, to apply what I learned, and to take responsibility for the consequences. I had to learn to fly, to surf these waves the way Billy did. That was how humans and animals thrived, by going beyond what they are taught, by paying attention to instinct, to feel, to experience

When I lost my wonder, the ability to ask questions disintegrated into questioning, doubting myself. When I stopped asking questions, I lost the ability to learn what no one else could teach me. When I learned only what others taught me, I lost what was unique about my experience, my skills, my talent. I lost myself.

In a world defined by self-help programs, I had discovered something deeper, more meaningful--self-education. Wide open possibilities that turned the freedom of choice into a search for the unknown, that transcended what was in front of me by creating endless degrees of freedom.

I came here year after year to remind myself of wonder, to strengthen it, to pursue the ideals that seem so cliché now—life, liberty, and happiness. Maybe Lindbergh idealized evolution making it sound more desirable, more kind than it was.

I had learned, was learning, however, that paying attention to this process worked as long as I took responsibility for it, as long I applied what I learned, and learned from the resulting experiences and data. I had seen with my own eyes that the most successful people, the happiest people, knew what Billy Pelican represented to me—that the best came not when we tried our hardest, but tried our best. The best results, the greatest performances, occurred when we rode the wind and the waves, when we embraced them instead of fought them.

The Most Important Lesson No One Ever Taught Me was that how I felt mattered in this process.

T. E. Lawrence, better known as Lawrence of Arabia, once described himself as "a standing civil war." I, too, was a soldier in this fight. I have come to understand that this standing civil war for me, for many people, begins in childhood when we are told that growing up means ignoring how we feel in the name of responsibility. The battle is sustained when we do everything we are supposed to do in life to fulfill those responsibilities, but find ourselves disconnected and unsatisfied. Life does not feel the way we thought it would. No one ever taught me about this battle, how to fight it, or how to triumph in it.

Lawrence described this dissonance in his "Seven Pillars of Wisdom:

We were fond together because of the sweep of open places, the taste of wide winds, the sunlight, and the hopes in which we worked. The morning freshness of the world-to-be intoxicated us. We were wrought up with ideas inexpressible and vaporous, but to be fought for. We lived many lives in those whirling campaigns, never sparing ourselves: yet when we achieved and the new world dawned, the old men came out again and took our victory to remake in the likeness of the former world they knew. Youth could win, but had not learned to keep, and was pitiably weak against age. We stammered that we had worked for a new heaven and a new earth, and they thanked us kindly and made their peace.[1]

By rekindling wonder, by asking questions of people who had won their standing civil war, I learned that how I felt not only mattered, but that paying attention to it *was* responsible. How I felt was data that allowed me to evolve, to make adjustments. In this way, I had lived my childhood dream. Like Billy Pelican, I found times that I could surf in my life, fly with the wind, and survive the Nor'easters that blew harshly into my face, impeding progress. It made me a better person. I had learned the difference between selfish momentary impulse and the purity of "feel."

My ability to feel was mine and mine alone. It was my personal source of data. It was the input of experience, human data my mind used to make decisions instead of settling for the intellectual choices

---

[1] T. E. Lawrence, Seven Pillars of Wisdom

others put in front of me. Poet Robert Frost wrote about two diverging paths, with one less taken by the multitudes. Two choices were too limiting for me. New waves appeared every few seconds and like Billy Pelican, I had learned to ride one at a time, to enjoy the ride, to trust how they felt to me. I understood what came to form the waves I found the most enjoyable and the most effective. I could predict where and when they appeared. And this? Well, it has made all the difference.

I turned my back to the waves and pushed forward, timing it so a wave caught me perfectly. I stuck my right arm straight out, a rudder steering me down the face of the wave into the perfect position. I was gliding forward and sideways with the wave as the curl loomed just behind me, then overhead. I pictured Billy adjusting to the subtleties of the wind as I adjusted to the idiosyncrasies of the wave. It gently deposited me on the shore and the smile crept back onto my face.

How I felt mattered. It was a lesson no one ever taught me, a lesson we could only learn on our own. It was a lesson that empowered me not only to win, but to hold onto that victory in the face of Lawrence's "old men." It was a lesson that allowed me to touch, to live my dream each and every day.

Chapter 1

Telling Your Story

I Feel Stuck

"I'm looking for Dr. Newburg. Do you know where I can find him?"

I turned to see an out-of-shape guy, mid 40's, leaning his head into the door of my office. He looked like one of those medical book pitchmen who parade through my office and waste my time.

"I'm Doug Newburg." I hate being called Dr. Newburg, especially because I work with real doctors. "Can I help you?" I pushed the chair away from my desk and rocked back.

"I thought you would be older. How old are you?"

I hear this all the time. "Never mind. I'm Bob Buchanan. I tried calling you, but you never seem to answer your phone, so I thought I would drop in. Some friends of mine heard you speak last week. They thought I should come talk with you."

No salesman. I wondered what he did for a living, and what he really cared about. I hoped they were the same thing, but I doubted it. I reached out to shake his hand. It was cold and clammy. He seemed nervous. I held onto his hand and put my left hand across it. He relaxed his shoulders and sighed.

"Let's take a walk," I suggested.

The hallways at the University of Virginia Hospital were atypical. The administrators were committed to bringing a sense of life to an inherently depressing place. Photographs of the Virginia countryside hung on the wall, reminders of healthier places beyond the bowels of the hospital. The doctors arrive before dawn and leave after dusk. These photos often serve as their only source of daylight.

Bob and I walked outside, past the serpentine walls surrounding the gardens that had begun the retreat for the onset of winter. We stepped through the archway and up to the Rotunda. The steps facing The Lawn, the original rooms at Thomas Jefferson's University, were my usual first meeting place with a client. The color dripped sparingly down the leaves in brown, yellow, and orange. The missing autumn splash of vibrant color reminded me of the dry summer. The mountains rose up behind Cabel Hall at the opposite end of The Lawn. Undergrads tossed Frisbees as their dogs cut across the turf like Barry Sanders, changing direction at full tilt. I smiled as I felt the athleticism of the dogs flow through me, taking me back twenty years.

The glorious scenery around us was powerless to disperse the dismal cloud that surrounded Bob. He was afraid of me, unsure of why he was here. He plopped down on the marble steps in his coat and tie. I sat next to him and leaned back on my elbow, turning my body to face him.

"So what do you want to talk to me about?" I asked.

"Well, as I said, several of my friends heard you speak and they thought you might be able to help me. They liked what you had to say."

A few weeks earlier, I had given a talk at The Darden Business School, part of the University. Actually, I ran more of a discussion among the people in the audience. We talked about making our lives better, about the struggle to create and maintain the life inside of us, and the cost of doing so.

"Why do you need my help?"

"I just feel stuck in my life. I have a good job, great family, and nice house. Still, it doesn't feel right. It's not what I thought it would be."

"What do you mean?"

"I don't know. That's the problem. I want to enjoy my life more." He paused. He sat forward and placed his face in his hands, his elbows on his knees. He looked beaten down. I thought he was going to cry. "I grew up thinking that if I had a good job and took care of my family, I would feel better about things than I do. I spend my life putting out fires that everybody else starts. My boss is always on me to do more. My wife wants me to spend more time with her and the kids. I want to do that, too, but I also want to do something just for myself."

I sat up and leaned towards him.

"What do you want to do for yourself?"

He raised his head and turned, looking me right in the eye. Anger and frustration were all over his face. His hands balled up into fists.

"That's just it. I don't even know what I would do. I just want to be free to do something for myself. I want to spend time with my family, and I want to do a good job at work, but I'm just spinning my wheels. I'm tired all the time. I'm out of shape. I played basketball in high school and intramurals in college. Man, I miss that. I was cocky. Now I feel like I don't have any confidence."

It was a familiar story. Check the societal boxes: degree, car, house, wife, kids. No matter where you are, who you are, you can turn into a maintenance man.

"You wouldn't be here if you didn't have any confidence."

"What do you mean?" He thought this was a trick, psychobabble. I suspected he wondered what he was doing here.

"What I mean is that if you didn't think you could do more or deserve more, you wouldn't be talking to me. You obviously think you can do something about it or you wouldn't be here. The real question is, "What do you do about it?""

"Okay, then what *do* I do?"

I lay back down on the steps. "The first thing you do is make yourself comfortable." He sat back. He looked ridiculous in his coat and tie. His white shirt gathered around his waist and his jacket seemed like it was going to burst a seam across the back. His face was red from the tightness of his collar and tie. "Let's talk a while and then you can decide if you want to work with me."

I reached up and touched the knot on his tie. "Take this thing off. Your coat, too. Tell me how you got to this point in your life. Start wherever you want. Just tell me your story."

"Everything?"

"Everything you think I should know about you."

He sighed and leaned forward again. He didn't see the point. He was afraid to look at the past; afraid of realizing he had wasted the last twenty years of his life. He sat silent for a few minutes, then gathered himself and took a few deep breaths. He was trying to trust me, but he wasn't quite ready.

"Alright. I grew up in a typical middle-class neighborhood. We lived pretty well, but nothing fancy. My dad made a decent living. My mom stayed home with my two brothers and me. We lived near a park that had some basketball courts and a baseball field and we were always playing sports." His face lit up and all of a sudden, he had a presence about him. He turned and looked right at me. His hands did as much of the talking as his voice did. His eyes grew wide.

"We played all day during the summer and after school during the year. Man, I loved that. We pretended we were the pros winning the NBA title or the World Series. That's what I remember most about being a kid. I could come and go and play. I had chores to do, but I always got up early to get those out of the way so I could play. My brothers and I would help each other so the work would get done. Our lives were about playing.

"I even liked school. I was a good student, one who didn't have to work hard to get good grades. I loved solving problems. When I was a teenager, my brothers and I used to work on cars. We loved figuring things out and fixing them. I have always had a natural curiosity about things."

As Bob talked he was energized, focused. He was telling me who he was as a kid, who he still wanted to be as an adult. That is what I look for in a person, that sense of involvement, of being oneself. I'm sure he didn't even notice how much he had changed just by remembering a time gone by, misplaced, but not lost. I knew I would be able to help him if he was willing to do the work.

Then Bob's story turned unpleasant. He slumped forward. His story lacked emotion. He skimmed over the details. His story telling turned into journalism. Flat, boring, sad.

Bob told me about messing around in college and being bored by the classes. College was a means to an end, a degree that led to a good job. He wanted a family, and knew he would be responsible for them. He wanted to provide for them. In his own words, he "wanted to be a man."

Bob described the last ten years of his life without emotion. He merely gave me the facts. The job he took because the company had good benefits and a decent salary. The sedan he drove. The minivan his wife drove. The work in the Technology Center of a huge mortgage company. The job that mostly entailed maintaining the current computer setup. He described the responsibility he felt in keeping things working. He grew more exasperated describing the day-to-day requirements of his job. People blaming him for crashes and lost earnings. His staff under-trained because of the fast pace growth of the computer field. He was merely maintaining the status quo technologically, but business demands growth. His company's goal was double-digit growth every year. "How can we keep doing that if nothing else in our department is allowed to grow?" Bob stated.

Bob was also responsible for choosing the equipment that they needed for the future. He said he never had time to deal with the future, because he was always fixing the present. The people he worked with were friendly, but incredibly busy. They never said, "Hi," to each other. They were just rushing around. They all had pagers that never quit beeping. He couldn't solve problems the way he wanted to because another new problem always pulled him away. His people were not given the training they needed to perform at a high level or to even keep up with their competition in the marketplace. That trapped them in their jobs. They lacked experience in the leading edge technology needed to compete for new jobs. Maintenance and administrative costs were kept down on purpose because they didn't look good to shareholders. All that mattered was the stock price. It was sad to listen to. Bob's innate curiosity for life had waned over the past ten years.

He didn't say much about his family except that everything he did was to keep them safe. He complained about not having the time to be with them. When he was there, he didn't have the energy to engage with them. He missed them emotionally, physically.

"My old man worked hard at the same job for 35 years. My mom took care of us, keeping us out of his hair. They were good parents, and they did the best they could. I loved them for that. I knew they wanted more out of life, but they hid it from us. My dad retired recently. He sits around the house. He doesn't know what to do without working. Sometimes he'll put on his coat and tie and just go walk. He seems so lost. We've tried to help him, but we don't know what to do. We worry about him. He won't travel, although my mom wants to, because he is afraid of outliving his money. He still feels responsible."

"Why is your dad important to your story?" I asked.

"I don't want that to happen to me. All the things I loved as a kid seem to be missing. There is no sense of play in our lives. My dad has lost his ability to play. I want to find mine again. I thought that was what retirement was about. "

"What keeps you from finding it?"

"I already told you. Everything I do is for someone else. I can't just forget my job or my family. I have a mortgage, car payments; college tuition is coming up. I can't turn my back on those things!" Anger swept into his voice. His eyes narrowed as he spun his head towards me in a non-verbal attack.

"If I asked how your life feels to you, what would you say?" I asked, ignoring his anger.

"I'd say I don't care about that touchy-feely stuff. It doesn't do any good. It just makes you weak, vulnerable."

"You said you wanted to talk to me because your life didn't feel the way you wanted it to. You sound pretty weak right now. You certainly sound vulnerable."

His body shook for a second. He covered his face with his hands. He braced himself, wiped his eyes, and took a deep breath.

"I don't want to talk about it."

"Let me ask you a couple of questions. When was the last time someone asked you if they could help you feel the way you wanted to feel?"

Bob laughed a sad laugh. When I talk to groups and ask that question, they laugh the same way.

"Never, right?"

"Right." Bob's head dropped again. I could tell he was wondering why such a question even mattered.

"Okay, does how you feel effect how you perform?" I asked.

He looked up, out into the distance.

"Of course it does," Bob said adamantly. I let the moment hang. Slowly a smile emerged. He sat straight up, his shoulders pushing back. He got it.

"No one has ever asked me that question before."

"Exactly. No one ever asked me either. I had to learn it on my own. Of course, how we feel effects how perform. How we live, too.

And if no one ever asks you how they can help you feel the way you want to feel, what does that tell you?"

"I have no idea."

"That feeling the way you want to feel, feeling the way that allows you to perform your best is your responsibility. I heard this over and over again in my interviews.

"Let me explain what I do and how I do it. Then the rest is up to you. The question is not really what you want. The question is what will you work for. We can sit here and fantasize all you want about how life should be. I want to know what you will do to get what you want. Did you ever have a teacher that really excited you, that challenged you and made you think?"

"Yeah. In high school. An English teacher, Mrs. Haynes. She was great."

"Why was she so great?"

"She made learning fun. She wasn't always telling us what we did wrong. She didn't worry about the grammar and sentence structure. I mean she made us work on those things, but she helped me understand why I was learning and how it related to me. She made me think about writing as a career. She wanted to know about me by how I related to the books we read. She wanted us to put our heart and soul into the things we wrote, the stories we told."

"That's how I want you to think about me. I am not here as a therapist. Did you have a psychologist who sat in Mrs. Haynes' class?"

"Of course not."

"Yet she still got you to look inside of yourself and to put that on paper, to process it?"

"Sure."

Bob was smiling as he talked about Mrs. Haynes. He remembered the freedom she gave him. He remembered how she inspired him to learn, to improve, to put his heart and soul into his work, onto the paper.

Enjoying Your Talent

I sat forward and rubbed my hands together. I'm always a little uncomfortable talking about myself. I certainly don't want to project myself as some great success story.

I consider myself successful, though, on my own terms. Every team, every organization I have been part of has enjoyed great success. I was rarely the star, but always knew I had a contribution to make. My high school basketball team went from years of losing seasons to district championships. My college team was one of the best in the country. I sold software for one of the best companies in the world. The University of Virginia where I received my degrees is one of the best institutions of higher learning in the world. In the Surgery Department, where I now work, we changed a difficult educational experience for medical students into an award winning learning environment.

I have seldom been the star or the prime player, but I have been around success all of my life. I have learned from the people around me. I have learned that every team needs role players. That is what my contribution has been. I consider myself successful in that function, because that is who I am. I did not become a role player by acquiescing, or by denying my own talents and dream. Being a role player allows me to live the way I want to live.

It is that experience of success that I share with people when I give talks, when I share my own story. Understanding that about myself was difficult and took years to understand. It is that process of understanding I wanted to impart to Bob.

"About ten years ago when I was in my later twenties, I realized, like you, that my life didn't feel the way I wanted it to. I sold software for a living and made decent money. I was married, owned a house, two cars, and we were headed towards a couple of kids. Then I came across a quote that changed my life. As he approached death at 35, Mozart said, 'I am finished before I have enjoyed my talent.' That really hit me. As a basketball player in college, I had finished playing before knowing how good I could be. In high school, I loved hoops more than anything, but I chose a college for all the wrong reasons. I wanted to play on television and play for a national championship, but the truth is I wasn't good enough. I hadn't worked smart enough or hard enough.

"When I read Mozart's words, I realized I was still headed down the wrong path to enjoy my talent, to enjoy myself. I went back to school to get my Ph. D., not for the degree, but because I wanted to learn how to enjoy my talent. It seemed reasonable to me that if I had talent and I enjoyed it, I would work hard and be productive enough to make a living.

"Early into the program I realized that the questions I had would not be answered by my pursuit of a degree. Then a conversation set me on the path I am still on. I was talking with a friend of mine, Dr. Gordon Davis, a veterinarian, and he told me that I should go find five people who live life the way I wanted to live. He said, "Don't worry about the things they have or what they do. Do they seem happy? Are they engaged in their lives?" I remember thinking: "Do they enjoy their talent?

"So that's what I did. I started with five people. Over the last ten years, I have interviewed more than 500 people. They are all successful, not only on society's terms, but also on their own terms. They are people I enjoy being around. All of them were willing to share their story. What they taught me was not just what they know, but how they know it."

Bob wasn't budging, sitting on the end of the step. His eyes told me he was excited.

"What I will share with you is how they live their lives, how they created their lives." I pointed across The Lawn and asked Bob, "What do you know about the University of Virginia?"

"Not Much. I went to Tech. I remember the basketball teams you played on. You guys were good. Ralph Sampson, Jeff Lamp. I don't remember you, though." Ouch.

"This Lawn was created as an "academical village." Thomas Jefferson's idea was that students learned as much from each other as they did in class. He wanted a place where life was about learning. He wanted a place that solved real problems. His idea was to create a place that developed leaders. The academical village has suffered over the years, but the idea is still sound.

"In a sense, I created my own "academical" community. The people I interviewed shared with me the things we don't learn in school or at work. They taught me about ideas and how to make them come to life in a responsible and useful way. My ideas. They taught me that performance at the most fundamental level is the creation and expression of ideas."

"I don't understand. What do you mean? That sounds too theoretical to me."

"Let me give you an example. You said you liked solving problems as a kid, right?"

"Right."

"But now you go to work and put out fires. Isn't putting out fires merely problem solving? What's changed? Why do you hate doing that now?"

"Because I'm doing it for everyone else. I'm solving problems that don't mean much to me. They just help me keep my job."

"Right. So in a sense you are merely expressing other people's ideas. Your talent is being used, but not to its fullest. And you don't enjoy it. Why did you love your English teacher so much? She gave you the problem and let you solve it from within. Your ideas, your words, your feelings. If she had just cared about grammar and sentence structure, you would've been bored."

"I get it."

"You got excited when you talked about procuring the equipment for the future. Do you have much say in that planning?"

"I have a say in the planning, but I don't have the time to carry it through to fruition. I like planning and implementing because it takes creativity and thought. My ideas matter. I see where you're going with this."

The sun was fading into the mountains. I had to finish calculating the grades for the third-year medical students. The Dean's office was growing impatient.

"That's enough for today. Let me know if you want to continue. If you do, I want you to call this number and ask for Jeff Rouse. Jeff was an Olympic swimmer who won three Gold Medals. I'll tell him you may be calling. Ask him to tell you his story. Then we'll meet again and you can tell me what you learned. Remember, this is not just about what you want in life, but also what you will work for."

"How can an Olympic gold medalist help me with what I'm going through? He's obviously very talented."

"I'm not sending you to Jeff because he has gold medals or because he has talent. I'm sending you to him because he is a good guy and has thought a lot about the same questions you're asking yourself. Trust me that when you meet him you'll know right away that he is a regular guy. Learn what you can from him. Before you go, I want to ask you a couple more questions. Did you have a dream as a kid?"

"Sure, I had a couple of dreams. First, I wanted to be a pro hoops player. When I realized I wouldn't be good enough, I thought about being a writer because of Mrs. Haynes. In the back of my mind I always thought I might have my own auto repair business."

"And what is your dream now?"

"Honestly, I can't say I have a dream. I am just trying to get by."

"If you didn't have a dream you wouldn't be here. You're just thinking about dreams in a not-so-useful way. Go call Jeff."

He looked at me in bewilderment. I know he was wondering why I ended our conversation this way. He shrugged it off. He trusted me. We stood and shook hands. This time his hand was warm and strong. He placed his left hand across mine and said, "Thanks. I will definitely be calling you."

I sat on the steps for a while longer. A long deep breath eased out of me. Listening to someone takes concentration. Maybe that's why people like Bob need someone to listen professionally. Good friends are harder and harder to hold onto in today's world, where the main business seems to be being busy. I felt I had listened to Bob.

I looked out over The Lawn and sat back against the steps. I must admit I get mildly disturbed at what people do to themselves and to each other. I include myself in this. I smiled. Listening to Bob made me realize how much I had changed over the past ten years. As an athlete, maybe even as a male, I had been taught that tougher is better. My high school coach taught me to fight, physically if need be, never to walk away. Ten years ago I would have listened to Bob and laughed. I would have told him to quit his whining, to be tough.

Being tough was the easy way to avoid what was real for me, the feeling that my birth mother didn't want me, that she gave me away. Sure, I'd heard all the reasons that what she was doing was best for me, that giving me away was the ultimate sacrifice for her to make. At an intellectual level, I respected her for that. But I still loved her and I missed her every day. Every failure, every rejection from a woman reminded me that she had left me in that hospital. Growing up, I just knew I was scared, yet I never examined what frightened me so. The fear usually turned into anger. What I wanted most in life was someone to be close to. The more I wanted it, the tougher I made myself, and the more I pushed people away.

I started toward the office, but turned instead to my car, deciding to do the grades the next day.

The pain I'd lived with all my life was her gift to me. The pain compelled me to do the work, to learn from others, to connect to what was best about me. Bob wasn't whining. He was listening to his own troubles. He was doing the work that most people just avoid.

Dear Douglas

The full moon illuminated my small town of Free Union. I could navigate the winding roads without headlights if I wanted to. As I pulled into my gravel driveway, several pairs of eyes looked at me from the woods. The frogs around the pond sang their nightly dirge. The dogs feverishly scratched at the door. I heard the familiar slap of the cats' swinging door as they headed inside and readied themselves for dinner.

I wondered what Bob went home to every night.

My mind wandered back to the time I decided my own life needed a change. It was triggered by an unfulfilling job and a boring marriage that eventually ended in divorce. As a result of the divorce, I finally looked into my emotional quagmire. My life was not terrible, but it also never felt right. It was hardly traumatic. My internal search began in earnest when I received a simple three-sentence letter from the foundling home in Washington, D. C.

Dear Douglas,

We have contacted your birth mother. She is not interested in a reunion. Your birth was a difficult time for her, and she does not want to relive it. As far as medical records the only thing she shared was that there was one case of diabetes in her family several generations ago.

Sincerely,

I don't remember the caseworker's name, but I have no trouble seeing the body of the letter in my mind. Reading the letter for the first time, I didn't acknowledge its impact. Looking back on it, though, I realized that I did what I always did. I hardened myself before I let it sink in. I just let it go. Or so I told myself.

I popped in a videotape of James Taylor performing in Boston. Of course he doesn't know it, but J.T. had helped me through some very difficult times over the past twenty years. I've seen him in concert 17 times. His lyrics are warm and comfortable, though not always happy and never sappy.

I pulled one of my thick, worn-out notebooks from the bookshelf. I plopped down on the couch to leaf through the words, the experiences I had collected over the years, looking for stories that might help Bob in his own life. My encyclopedia of stories empowered me with the knowledge of similar experiences successfully navigated by others. I am a collector of stories and experiences, just like someone who collects stamps or coins, although my collection seems far more useful, at least to me.

As I began to read, my dog, Righteous, jumped onto the couch, stepped on my groin, and placed his head into my lap. Riding bikes on Afton Mountain several years earlier, my friend Curt Tribble and I were confronted by twelve puppies parading out into the street in Disney-like fashion. We continued on our way, but returned to the scene later to ask if we could buy any of them. The runt of the litter was trampled into the muddy floor of their pen by his siblings. He looked up as if to say, "Get me out of here!" Tested, but not beaten, he fought to get to his mother's milk, each time pushed away by the little black feet of his brothers and sisters. He waited his turn, then took his time as the others dispersed. Maybe that was why I chose him first.

When I asked the owner if I could have a couple of the puppies, he said, "You can have all twelve." The owner, Sammy, was a strong black man. His powerful chest and oak-like arms told me he worked hard with his hands for a living. He probably thought it was silly that we were out exercising for fun. His fifty-plus year old hands brought me to my knees when we shook. The puppies were an accident, mutts, All-American dogs. Sammy pointed out the father across the street.

"That's Buck. He doesn't look too happy with you all eyeing his pups."

Buck stood erect, chest out, ears pointed. Buck was also a mutt. He looked like he was mostly shepherd, but with long fur.

"You know mutts make the best pets," Sammy continued. "They're smart. Shoot, you see these rich people spend all this money on purebreds and they're just dumb. They don't know enough to lick butter off a hot piece of bread. But you give me a mutt, that's a righteous dog." Hence, the name Righteous.

Righteous always needs to be touched. He sleeps with me every night and is always right at my feet when I 'm home. Jazz, Righteous's sister, is far more independent and distant. Righteous eventually outgrew Jazz into a handsome 70 pound All American mutt. I love Jazz just as much, but I seem to understand Righteous. Jazz merely represents my difficulty in understanding women. I can love her unconditionally, but I have no idea what she wants. As Righteous and I sat on the couch, Jazz hid under the coffee table waiting for a cat to wander by, when she'd pounce and chase them out the cat door.

Asking Useful Questions

My seven-speaker stereo was in full voice; J.T. sounded like the young cowboy in the song: down in the canyon, alone, but not lonely, thinking back on the women he'd loved. On the tape, the camera panned the audience, catching several people smiling and crying simultaneously, as if a cobweb-covered box full of memories had spilled open. A contradiction of loving and losing. The inability to separate one from the other, as our life rushes through our mind's eye. I know better now. These feelings belong together, commingled into my own tapestry, a mosaic only I can understand as a whole. Deciphering my own life was a purposeful quest, a conscious choice to do something about my feelings, about what I wanted in life. I chose to do the work. Was Bob willing to do the work?

In doing it on my own, I was in a sense in a different place than Bob. I had no guidelines other than Dr. Davis' suggestion that I find five people to talk to. What were they supposed to tell me? Were they supposed to give me the answers? I had struggled with what questions to ask them. I didn't know what I didn't know. There was something uncomfortable about talking to these successful people as I began.

My ignorance, however, turned out to be a blessing. I simply asked them to tell me how they got where they were. Most of them shared willingly, some of them talking for hours on end. As they talked, I locked onto their words, their movements. I listened without trying.

Questions burst out of me. Why had they chosen the life they had? Why were they willing to work so hard? What role did others play in their lives, in their successes and failures? How did they hold onto their lives despite tremendous obstacles? What was the cost of fighting for themselves? What was the result?

When I work with people, I often ask them to go find people in their lives that live the way they want to live and learn from them. I understand the fear, the uncertainty my clients feel in doing this simple task. I remembered feeling that same fear, and asking the same questions. Why would these people talk to me? What if I ask a dumb question? Won't they think something is wrong with me? I knew Bob was having these thoughts as he sat at home staring at the phone, the receiver in his right hand, the left hand gripping the phone, sweat on his palms, like the first time a guy calls a girl for a date. I once called a girl so many times and hung up without talking, her father had the number changed. Thank God they hadn't invented Caller ID back then.

I called Jeff Rouse and told him Bob would likely be calling. I asked Jeff to answer only the questions that Bob asked, but to answer them completely. Bob would have to listen for the next question, not simply for the answer. Jeff understood that this was a learning process for Bob. Bob had to learn how to learn, how to ask the right questions. *Living life is about asking useful questions, and then finding the answers for yourself.* In the medical field, students are taught that the specific knowledge they acquire in treating patients will change every five years. Our task as educators is to teach them to ask the right questions. As we grow older, our questions remain the same, but the answers differ because we need different things at different times of our lives.

Jeff said, "No problem." Actually, Jeff enjoyed this process. He would learn something from Bob. Jeff once told me that learning to articulate his own process made it more useful to him. Telling his own life experiences out loud gave them meaning for his present and his future. That was why I had asked Bob to tell me his story. We can learn a lot from others, but we also have to know how we got where we are. We need to undo some beliefs, to unlearn some habits. We need to undo the structure built around our own processes. Telling my story to myself was a way to start living my own process, and to shed the structure that had protected me, but was now too limited. It limited me to the strength of the structures around me. Saying out loud that I was scared, that I felt a sense of loss for my birth mother made it real, and in a small way gave me some control over it. Jeff had a similar experience relative to swimming.

In telling himself his own story between the Olympics of 1992 and 1996, Jeff identified his process as a person and as a swimmer. He abandoned the structure that had outlived its purpose. Jeff grew up in Fredericksburg, VA and is as close to the All-American kid as I have ever known. He was a world-record holder in the 100-meter backstroke and was ranked No. 1 in the world for 8 years.

I met Jeff right after the 1992 Olympics in Barcelona. A mutual friend set me up to interview him. I had no idea that interview would lead Jeff and me to become great friends. I wanted to know what Jeff knew, and how he had learned it. In Jeff's mind he had lost in the Olympics by placing second. He was devastated by the loss. This showed in the first interviews I did with him. We struggled to talk about his experiences. We knew we had similar feelings about sport, about competition, and about life. The problem was that language seemed inadequate to describe these things. In spite of this inauspicious beginning, we connected enough to want to continue to talk with each other. The conversation is never-ending.

Knowing Why, Not Just How

I refocused on helping Bob. In my notebook of meaningful stuff, I came across a letter that my friend, Curt Tribble, had received from a former teacher, Jim Skinner from Presbyterian College in South Carolina. Dr. Tribble and I work together at the Medical School overseeing the educational aspects of the Surgery Department. Jim had visited us at UVa. and listened to the philosophy we employ to educate the students and residents. Jim wrote to us and included a section of a speech his brother had given recently. I'll never forget the first time Curt showed it to me. We were preparing for orientation of the students. Curt pulled out the letter and said he wanted to read it to the students, but didn't think he could make it through it. It was too emotional. I took the letter from Curt and said I would read it to the students. I read through it, handed it back to Curt and said, "You're on your own," as a tear formed in the corner of my eye. Curt made it through fine, his low tone of voice making it that much more dramatic for the students:

"In the course of trying to persuade my father to go to Italy with me, I gave him a book. The book was titled 'The Architecture of the Italian Renaissance' by Peter Murray. In the introduction to the book, the author eloquently describes the sources of Renaissance architecture and makes the connections to the history and philosophy and religion of the times.

My father was never an avid reader, but one day about seven years ago, I sat with my father in his living room. As I was reading the newspaper, my father sat down in his rocking chair beside me and began to read. After several minutes I looked up and was greatly surprised to see there were tears in his eyes, tears rolling down his cheeks. I said , 'Dad what's wrong?' He looked up at me and in a voice almost anguished, he said to me: 'Why didn't I ever know these things? Why did I never learn this?'

He went on to explain that, at Georgia Tech, where he had gone to school to learn to become an architect, all they had ever taught him was how to design a building, how to build a building. They had never encouraged him to look beyond this, to explore the whys and wherefores of the architecture, to probe beneath the surface of technique or to make those vital connections between architecture and religion and philosophy and history. Just how to build and nothing more. And in that moment, there was such a sense of loss, of profound sadness at my father's realization of what had been missing all those years laboring in his profession, sweating to meet deadline after deadline after deadline."

I had decided to give the letter to Bob because of the story he told of his father. I pictured Bob's father walking the street in his jacket and tie, wondering what to do with himself after retirement. I could see how that would scare Bob so much. The question loomed heavy. What does someone do to avoid such a fate? I thought of Bob interviewing Jeff, of what the poet William Blake called the "minute particulars" that shape our lives. Each day, we have opportunities to take control of our lives, of our own fate. We need to look for them, to observe and participate, to effect change. Bob's first goal was to observe the minute particulars of his life.

My own father retired several years ago from the federal government. He went through a similar period as Bob's father. He didn't really know what to do with himself. He had been good at his job in the Department of Housing and Urban Development. He had received numerous awards, and he was highly ranked for a non-political appointee. But when he retired, we worried about him because he seemed uninspired. He still had so much to offer the world, but he seemed uninvolved. Eventually, I asked him to help me write. That gave him new life, and he attacked the assignment passionately. He got to the point that he was pressing me to catch up with him.

As we worked together I realized something about him that I had seen in so many others, especially from his generation. He was used to working for others, for his family. Now, any work he had to do was strictly for himself. He and my mom had invested wisely. My mother was still working and he was waiting for her to retire. He had planned his financial retirement, but not his emotional retirement from work, or at least working for others.

When my mother retired a year later, they began to travel, to remodel their house, to really live. Arthur Ashe once said that physical retirement is a decision, but emotional retirement takes it own course. My father had separated from the physical requirements of going to work each day, but he was having trouble living with the freedom in his life he had earned, that he had created through wise investment and hard work. In a sense, it was this process that Bob wanted to begin while he still worked.

Bob knew the rules of the societal games. He played by them and had a good foundation to start from. He had a loving family, a good job, and some money in the bank. Bob wanted to enjoy these things, to experience them the way he wanted, to use them to improve the quality of his life and the lives of those around him.

I laughed out loud. What did I know about societal rules? I had been a rebel from day one. Not a pot smoking, break-the-law kind of rebel. I was always responsible, but I had rebelled by not allowing people or institutions to determine my fate in life. I wanted to be myself no matter where I was or what I was doing. When I did those things, I usually performed well. When I tried to conform, I became lost and confused and had no foundation on which to rely. I never had any great ambition in life other than to do what I loved. As a kid, it was obvious what I loved: playing, serious go-to-the wall playing. As an adult, though, it became difficult to find the place I could really play and be myself. That had been my task, to find the things I loved doing and to find the things that were an expression of who I was in a productive, responsible manner.

The most important lesson that no one ever taught me was what I learned from the many successful people I interviewed. That lesson was that how I feel matters. I learned that how I feel affected everything I did—how I performed, how I lived. I learned that feeling the way I wanted to feel was my responsibility... and my freedom. Malcolm Gladwell said it best in an article he wrote for *The New Yorker*. That article was called *The Physical Genius*[2], an article about high-level performers from a variety of fields. Gladwell suggested that the foundation of their genius was that they had "found something that, on some profound, aesthetic level, made them happy."

This echoed what I had heard in my interviews—that these people reached high levels of performance, of living, because they found and did things that made them happy as they were doing these activities. They collected data about how they felt, some more systematically than others, but it was data collection nonetheless. The goal with Bob was to help him discover for himself a process for collecting the meaningful and data that was his and his alone.

This also led me to another subtle but important distinction—between *feelings* and *feel*. Seemed to me that we had turned the word "feelings" into almost a negative word, one that meant emotional baggage or issues. The word "feel," however, had maintained its vigor. The people I interviewed talked about how they felt more than about their feelings. How we feel is data that can lead us into different directions because how we feel is more than the emotional response to things in our lives. It distinguishes between momentary impulses that result from childhood experiences or experimentation and how we want to feel in the long run, every day, day after day. It allowed me to see that happiness is more than an emotion. Happiness is a feel, a personal experience. *Happiness is feeling the way we want to feel.*

I wondered why no one had ever taught me these things. Sure, people said do what you love, but that was too specific and relied on knowing what you loved doing. But finding and doing the things that made you happy, that made you feel the way you wanted to feel, made sense and seemed within anybody's grasp, within my grasp. That was resonance with a small "r." That was where we all start—paying attention to how we feel one moment, one day at a time. If we're diligent, if we take responsibility for how we feel, we string those experiences together into a career and a life that resonates within us. We feel the way we want to feel. It is a process that begins with acknowledging that how we feel matters. It is a process that is nurtured by observation and experience.

---

[2] Malcolm Gladwell, The Physical Genius (The New Yorker, August, 1999).

Chapter 2

Easy Speed

Dreams and Goals

Bob burst into the office without knocking. He was early and eager. He stood in the doorway. I assumed he wanted to go outside again. It was a beautiful day, mid 60's and sunny, so I agreed. We walked out to my Jeep Wrangler and hopped in, top down. Bob was busting. He wanted to talk, but I cranked the stereo and we headed out to my house 15 minutes away. The blue sky seemed to bleed into the mountain that rose up from behind my house.

"Where are we going?" Bob asked.

"See that triangular mountain. We're going to sit at its base. That's where I live." Buck Mountain looked closer than it was. Bob grew impatient and started squirming in his seat.

"Rouse was nothing like I expected. I figured a gold medalist would be intense. He was a nice guy, laid back."

I ignored Bob for the moment as we drove through Free Union. We pulled into the gravel driveway as my dogs and cats came running. The dogs didn't wait for Bob to dismount. They were in his lap as soon as the car stopped. He fended them off and hopped down. He was in jeans and a polo shirt this time. He seemed more comfortable.

We headed to the lake and said goodbye to my dogs, Jazz and Righteous. I heard their collars beeping, warning them to stop before they ran into the invisible fence. They sat and panted. They'd be there when we came back. It was lunchtime and they really didn't have anything better to do.

Buck Mountain rose out of a small lake into the blue sky. We sat on the shore my neighbor had cleared with his tractor. The fish swam close to check us out. We could see several feet deep into the water, the perch hovering just out of our reach.

"This is awesome. I wish I could live near something like this."

"Why can't you?"

"Never really thought about it."

"So what did you learn from Jeff?"

"Where do you want me to start?"

"What surprised you the most about what he said?"

"I was surprised at how low-key he was. I didn't expect it. Then I was surprised at how nice he was and that he would take time to talk to me."

"Why do those things surprise you?"

"I don't know. Television makes these guys out to be super human. I didn't believe you when you said that I could learn something from him. I figured he had no idea what it was like to be me, yet he understood exactly what I was feeling."

"What makes you say that?"

"Well, the best way to explain it would be to talk about a distinction he made. He distinguished between a dream and a goal. He said a dream is the way you want to feel. It is an internal quality, something you feel."

"Something touchy-feely?"

Bob laughed. "Yeah, something touchy-feely. When he told me his dream, I knew exactly what he was talking about. I had felt it myself. I understood that it was a feeling, something inside of him. He called it Easy Speed. He described it as going 90 to 100 percent of your maximum speed, but with 80 percent effort. He said that was why he swam. He wanted to find Easy Speed in his life and in whatever he does. He really believes he can do that. He actually expects to feel Easy Speed every day in one form or another. He described how he had felt it when he worked on his house or fixed his car or taught little kids. Easy Speed was a way of life, not just something he felt when he swam. It sounded wonderful. I have felt that before myself."

"Really. When?"

"Mostly when I was a kid. I have felt it at work at times also. I'm working on something and all of a sudden the day has flown by. Most of the time I feel it when I have a project that I am left alone on or when the team is really working together. If I tried to describe Easy Speed to someone who was not involved in sports, I would say it is when things are meaningfully efficient. We are working on something important to us, we are doing it well, and we move at a good pace. We don't worry about time or eating or taking calls. We are all trying to solve the problem."

"You mean put out fires?"

"Sometimes."

"I thought you hated that."

"I do most of the time."

"Well, what's the difference between when you hate it and when you feel Easy Speed?"

"I'm not sure I know what you mean."

"What did Jeff say about training for Easy Speed? Did he feel like he could make it happen more often than not?"

"Oh, yeah. He said the cool thing in Atlanta in '96, when he won the gold, was that he made Easy Speed happen. It was fun watching him talk about it. He got excited and energized. He said he could feel Easy Speed sitting in the chair and talking about it."

Bob looked out over the lake. He was relaxed. Some geese flew overhead catching Bob's eye. His whole body followed their flight as they skimmed the surface of the water, made a quick turn, and disappeared over Buck Mountain. They never broke formation. Above the mountain a single hawk floated on a thermal. The hawk rose into the sky and then dropped back down, changed its angle, and rose again. Bob pointed and whispered, "Easy Speed."

The Process

"Teach me what you learned from Jeff," I said.

"How?"

"Tell me what you learned that applies to your life. What did he share with you that is useful to you?"

His eyes narrowed and he looked down at the water. He knew he had learned something useful, but articulating it was still difficult.

"I'm not sure how to do that. I know I learned a lot, but not well enough to share it in any useful way."

He reached into his pocket and pulled out a large, crumpled, white napkin.

"Jeff showed me something he called the process. He said you developed it from your interviews. He told me that the process you developed put a language to the way he had lived most of his life. Until the process had been articulated, he felt that much of his life just happened by accident. The Process allowed him to make much of his life happen on purpose or, what did he say, by design."

"Explain this process to me."

"I'm not sure I fully understand it."

"That's okay. Try anyway."

Bob flattened the napkin, smoothing out the edges. He was stalling more than worrying about its condition.

I glanced down and saw a hand-drawn version of the process I use to teach people. There were notes all over it. How many bar napkins had I drawn this on before? The simplified process looks like this:

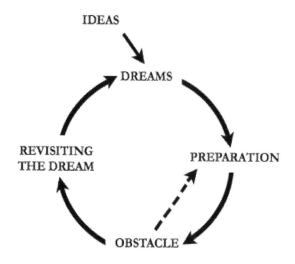

THE RESONANCE MODEL

Bob was silent, not quite sure where to begin.

"I'll start with ideas. That is where you and I began last time we met. *Ideas are the catalyst for any action or reality.* Anything we do seems to begin with an idea. Getting a job, making money, getting married, playing hoops, anything that we form in our minds that might lead to an action can be termed an idea."

The concept of an idea is simple to me. Anything that crosses our mind, that we pause to consider, that we might want to take action on, is an idea. Bob seemed to understand this. He accepted the simplicity of ideas. So many people make this harder than it is. The Oxford English Dictionary references Locke and Descartes in the definition of an idea, they describe an idea as: "whatever is in the mind and directly present to the cognitive consciousness: that with which one thinks, feels, or fancies; the immediate object of thought or mental perception." The beauty of ideas is their serendipitous nature. We are free to have ideas. In fact, we have them without trying. We are free to choose which ideas we will act on and which ideas we will discard. Life is a never-ending series of ideas.

Safety, Security, Acceptance.

Bob looked at me for confirmation. I didn't respond. He continued with a bit more confidence. As he talked he seemed to pay less attention to what I thought.

"Looking back on my life, I have had a lot of ideas that were externally driven. I did the things people thought were right, or things I was told to do. The more I did that, the fewer ideas I had on my own. I merely waited for others to formulate their ideas, and then I put them into action. Jeff described how that happened to him in the 1992 Olympics. He got angry talking about it. Other people convinced him that nothing he accomplished in swimming would matter if he didn't win a gold medal. That's ridiculous. He was a world record holder and a world champ, but he went into the '92 Olympics believing that if he didn't win a gold medal, he would have wasted his entire life in swimming. I can't imagine how much pressure he must have felt."

"So how does that apply to you?"

"I'm not sure yet. I think what you and Jeff would say is that I am putting too much pressure on myself, because all of my actions are based on the ideas of others. I spend all my time doing what others want, or at least what I think they want."

"Why do you think you do that?"

"Safety. Security. Acceptance."

"So you are really doing these things for others, because you want to feel a sense of security, of being accepted?"

"I guess that's right. I really do care what others think of me. I'm scared of failing."

"And do you feel safe? Do you feel accepted?"

"Not at all. In fact, I feel exactly the opposite. I'm only as good as the previous day at work or my latest paycheck. I feel like I'm always taking a test. Not only do I not know the answers, I don't even know the questions."

"So you spend your life answering questions that you don't know. The target keeps moving and the way you feel is dependent on how well you do on the test."

"Exactly."

"If you could choose how you want to feel everyday, what would those feelings be?"

"Well..." He paused. "That's a tough question. I'll have to think about it. It has been so long since I felt like myself that I can't answer that right away."

"Tell me about the next part of the process. The dream part," I prompted Bob.

"That was where Jeff distinguished between the dream and a goal. That distinction is difficult for me to accept. I've always thought of a dream as a tangible object that might be just out of my reach. I never really thought about a dream as being different from an ultimate goal. I stopped dreaming a long time ago, and just went from one goal to another. I usually reach my goals."

"How does it feel when you achieve your goals?"

"It feels pretty good. At work, we have to state our goals every year and I have met every one of them. It feels good to achieve something. The tough part is that as soon as I reach it, I can't really enjoy it, because I have to go after another goal."

"How about the procedure you go through to achieve the goals, the downtime between achievements? How does that feel?"

"Like drudgery. I keep thinking to myself I can't wait until I reach it. There are usually some other incentives attached to the goals. For example, to a large extent, the number of complaints we get is a measure of our unit's ineffectiveness, our failure rate. Our goals are often to minimize the number of complaints over a given time period."

Bob had some energy in his voice as he talked. He was proud of the fact that under his watch, the number of complaints had decreased significantly. He went on to say, though, that the better they were, the higher the expectations became. He felt that his job was more about avoiding punishment than about growth. As they were rewarded for fewer complaints, he saw people taking fewer risks. When he had taken the promotion, he thought he was positioning himself to be on the cutting edge of technology and to help his company move into the next millennium. He was excited as he talked about the possibilities. Then reality set in again. His voiced weakened.

"I think I took this job for the right reasons. It sounded like a great opportunity, but basically all we're doing is avoiding mistakes."

"Why do you think that?"

"Because all of our goals are based on eliminating downtime. We are judged by how well we avoid mistakes. Implementing new programs or technologies increases the number of complaints we get, in the short term."

"Who judges that?

"My boss."

"Has he said that specifically to you?"

"No."

"If he came to you and asked you what you want, do you think you could explain it in a way he could understand?"

"He would never ask that."

"I didn't ask you that. If he did ask, could you tell him?"

"Yes. No. I'm not sure."

"So if you don't know what you want, how can you hold him accountable for not giving you what you want. You don't know yourself. You haven't done the work to figure out what you really want. If an opportunity came along you'd miss it."

"I thought you were going to help me feel better."

"That's what we're headed towards, but this takes some real work. Remember I asked you what you would work for, not just some fantasy of what you'd like. The process is actually very simple, but it is difficult to do. It takes commitment, but you have to know what you're committing to first. That is why the dream stage exists. The task is to figure out what you want, how you want to feel, and what you will work for."

I Don't Have A Dream

Bob sat silently for a second. His head dropped as he struggled to tell me what he was feeling.

"I don't think I have a dream. I mean there is nothing I really want that I don't have."

"And yet you are still scared, vulnerable, unfulfilled."

"Yeah."

"If I asked you again how you'd like life to feel everyday, do you think you could answer that better now than last time?"

"Sure. I mean I want to feel different things at different times. But for the most part, I know how I'd like to feel."

"Then you have a dream."

"That's not a dream. A dream is like having a million dollars or winning some championship."

"That's one idea of a dream. Given how you feel about your life, would you say that's a useful idea? Does having a dream that you won't work for or don't think you will ever get make you feel better or worse?"

"Sometimes when I daydream, I can escape and it feels pretty good. Most of the time, though, I just feel like a failure because I know I won't achieve those things."

"So your idea of what a dream is, isn't useful to you. In fact, it sounds destructive."

"Okay. Yeah. Now I really feel bad."

"Hang in there. What did Jeff tell you about his experience relative to dreams?"

"When his dream was to win a gold medal, he felt like he drained himself trying to win one. He lost confidence. He worried about things he couldn't control, and worried about what other people thought. He swam to win the gold so he wouldn't let other people down."

"Sound familiar?"

A sheepish grin crept onto his face.

"What about the '96 Olympics?" I asked.

Bob sat forward; his hands began to dance as he talked. "He took some time to remember why he loved swimming. He went back to Easy Speed. He knew that the races in which he swam well, he felt Easy Speed. He knew he couldn't control winning, but he felt he could make Easy Speed happen most of the time. He thought back to '92 and what things affected him. In 1996 he took more control over his experience. He created a better environment to allow Easy Speed to happen."

"And what did happen?"

"He felt Easy Speed AND he won the gold medal. I think I'm beginning to understand. But I don't think Easy Speed is my dream. Maybe it is. But I don't know how to make it happen."

"What did Jeff tell you about how he learned this? Remember I told you to pay attention to how he knew what he knew, not just what he knew."

"I kept that in mind as we talked. I asked him how he knew things, how he learned what he needed to know. He said that he stopped making statements about how he was supposed to be, and began making observations about who he was and what was really important to him. He said that he realized his family would love him no matter how well he swam. He took the risk of telling the people closest to him what he needed from them: support, freedom, and understanding of what he was going through. He needed them to help him get away from all the hype of swimming and of the Olympics. That took a lot of pressure off of him. He stopped talking to the media, and he anticipated things that would cause him to lose his focus on Easy Speed. He thought back on his life as a swimmer, and he made observations about what made him feel Easy Speed, even when he was just sitting and thinking."

Five Useful Questions

"So now you know what you need to do?" I asked Bob.

"I guess so. But how do I observe myself?"

"People do it in different ways. I usually give them a tape recorder and ask them to talk into it every night and describe how they felt that day. Sometimes I just give them a bunch of beads to carry around. When they feel the way they want to feel, I ask them to connect one more bead to the chain. At night I ask them to make observations about those feelings."

"That seems too simple."

"I told you this is simple, but you'll be hard pressed to do it. I'll leave you with five questions to think about, to make observations about. I want you to process them every night for the next two weeks and then we'll talk again. The questions are:

1. How do you want to feel everyday or about your life in general?

2. When, where, and around whom do those feelings happen?

3. What gets in the way of those feelings or takes them away?

4. How do you get those feelings back?

5. What are you willing to work for?

"Try to answer those questions, and then we'll talk again in two weeks. To be clear, you are just making observations about what happens. Don't pressure yourself to make certain feelings happen, or to hold onto them. We'll get there. For now, we just want to figure out what you want, and what you might be willing to work for. Alright?"

Bob nodded. He still doubted the process as most people did. The idea of a dream being about how we feel each day seemed weak. I could tell he thought there had to be more to it.

The foundation of the process lies in the power of an idea that captures our attention. As we grow up, we rarely spend time focusing on our feelings. My belief is that most of our actions are built on a tacit knowledge of the consequences of those actions. If we undertake a specific activity, we can predict how we'll feel most of the time. We don't take control of that process to feel the way we want to. We deal with the feelings after we complete a task, leave a relationship, or just head home from work. The feelings we want in those post-activity moments are the feelings of escape. We stop wanting to feel anything at all. We numb ourselves to life. We numb ourselves to who we are. Even the best of us dread certain activities that we must do.

The difference between a dream and an idea is simply one of commitment. The people I interviewed committed themselves to the feelings of engagement, of fulfillment, of connection with others, and the experience of the purest elements of themselves. That is the dream. They pay attention to those experiences that inherently allow them to engage the best of themselves, and they invest in those experiences and in themselves. They do the work. Psychologist William James description seems appropriate:

It is, in one word, an idea to which our will applies itself, an idea which if we let it go would slip away, but of which we will not let go. Consent to the idea's undivided presence, this is the effort's sole achievement. Its only function is to get this feeling of consent into the mind. And for this there is but one way. The idea to be consented to must be kept from flickering and going out. It must be held steadily before the mind until it fills the mind. The idea must be given a quiet hearing.[3]

I read James as I worked on my dissertation. In his *Principles of Psychology*, he articulated what I was seeing in the people I interviewed, the commitment to an idea:

...who hears the small voice unflinchingly, and who, when the death-bringing consideration comes, looks at its face, consents to its presence, clings to it, affirms it, and holds it fast, in spite of the host of exciting mental images which rise in revolt against it and would expel it from the mind. Sustained in this way by a resolute effort of attention, the difficult object erelong begins to call up its

---

[3] William James, Psychology: The Briefer Course (Indiana: University of Notre Dame Press, 1985).

own congeners and associates and ends by changing the disposition of the man's consciousness altogether.[4]

The dreams of youth give way to the responsibilities of adulthood and we are challenged to hold onto our own ideas, to use our imagination, to give our own ideas "a quiet hearing." The values and beliefs of those around us shape our internal world, and we lose sight of the feelings we loved as children. Our educational processes are based more on learning and memorizing the ideas and thoughts of those who preceded us, than on discovering our true selves and engaging our own ideas and experiences.

What I have learned, is to understand at my core what draws me to an activity, to a person, to a lifestyle. Why am I interested in something? Why do I want to learn about something? The more I feel engaged, the more I want to feel engaged and fulfilled. It is dynamic. There is no final goal or outcome. Paraphrasing James and Pirsig, I have my own ideas, observe my experience of those ideas, and cling to those that engage me. That is the dream.

In working with people, I run the risk of having them try simply to follow the description of this process, to imitate it. My goal is to expose people to themselves so they can find their own processes, to have their own ideas, and to find the most meaningful and engaging ways of expressing those ideas: to **live** the process.

As Bob and I walked to the Jeep, I handed him a single sheet of paper.

"What's this?" he asked.

"Something from Walt Whitman, the poet," I replied. "I want you to think of the process as an introduction to yourself. We'll use it to help you discover more about who you are and what you want from your life. Ultimately, you will discover how to live the life you want, and it might look nothing like this. But you need to know more about yourself first. The worst thing you could do is to imitate what I'm teaching you, because then you are simply replacing one structure with another. Structures suck the life out of processes."

Neither of us spoke as I drove Bob back into town. Bob looked at the poem then looked up, and back again to the poem:

---

[4] Ibid.

Stop this day and night with me and you shall origin of all poems,

You shall possess the good of the earth and s millions of suns left,

You shall no longer take things at second or third hand...nor look through the eyes of the dead...nor feed on the spectre in books,

You shall not look through my eyes either, nor take things from me,

You shall listen to all sides and filter them from yourself.

Not I, not anyone else, can travel that road for you,

You must travel it for yourself.

It is not far...it is within reach

Perhaps you have been on it since you were born, and did not know

Perhaps it is everywhere on water and on land.

Shoulder your duds, and I will mine, and let us hasten forth:

Wonderful cities and free nations we shall fetch as we go. [5]

As I drove Bob back into town, he thought about the poem from Whitman, and enjoyed the view, the music, and the speed of the wind as it pushed through my Jeep. He hung his leg over the side where I had removed the door. The Goo Goo Dolls were cranking. I drove on instinct, by rote. Working with Bob reminded me of so many things I had done in my own life. It is still easy for me to forget to observe everything. They tell you to stop and smell the roses, but they don't tell you what is most important is finding your own scent. The key for me had been to observe what I felt when things happened to me, good or bad.

I dropped Bob off at the medical school. His hair had flown in every direction, but he had this satisfied smile on his face. Jeeps are fun. He climbed out, said he would be in touch, and sauntered away.

---

[5] Walt Whitman, Leaves of Grass (New York, The Penguin Group).

I suddenly was aware of a visceral feeling in my chest. When I operated best, when I enjoyed my life the most, when I made the best decisions, that's where I felt it. In earlier years, no matter what was happening to me, the visceral impact would always end up in the same place, in my stomach. When something great happened to me, I enjoyed it until I was alone. Then a grabbing pain hit my stomach, as I realized I didn't have anyone to share it with. Similarly, if something bad happened, I felt that pain in my stomach, this time from failure or rejection.

When I played sports, though, the visceral feeling was usually in my chest, a feeling of being bigger, stronger, more connected, unthreatened. So part of my dream was to enjoy the good feeling in my chest, not my stomach, lower back, or head. I wanted to feel this throughout my life, not just in sports.

Making Observations

When I send people off to observe themselves, they walk out of the office full of doubt that there *are* good moments in their lives. They think observing themselves will be easy, because so few good things happen to them. Invariably, they call me several days later and want to talk about how differently they are seeing their lives. It is actually easy to get somebody started doing this. The tough part is to help them do it long enough to make it a habit or a way of life.

I rocked back in my chair. The changes in my life started with the observations of my story, a look at my past. I needed to know more about myself, about the times I really enjoyed life. When were those times? What were the experiences? Who were they around? What made those people different?

I headed back to Buck Mountain. A swath of sky and cloud merged with the green mountains ahead of me. The clouds were a spectacular orange fading into pink. The sun was behind the mountains, the sky dark, but intensely blue. It was as if someone was standing in the valley splashing paint up onto the clouds.

I love living in the small town of Free Union, because I never get stuck in traffic. Occasionally, the random horse trailer or tractor will slow me down, but that is different. Traffic vexes me because it forces me to change my rhythm. Looking back, when I figured out what I wanted to feel every day, I realized that it was rhythm. When I run, when I shoot a basketball, when I write, when I work with someone, I am always looking to uncover a certain rhythm. Traffic is dissonant.

There is rarely a rhythm to traffic. Go fast, slow down, wait 20 minutes with no control or certainty to how long each small forward progression will be. I would rather drive twenty miles out of the way to avoid traffic, if I can maintain a rhythm.

That discovery led to other simple things. When I am in traffic on a highway and a line of cars is merging, I realized that letting someone merge feels a lot better than trying to box someone out. In the grocery store, people stand in line and complain about long lines, yet don't even think about bagging their own groceries. If there is a lone cashier, I can maintain the rhythm I want by bagging my own groceries. When I drive through town, it feels better to let pedestrians cross the street than ignore them. I make it my own idea. I adapt it into my rhythm, into my life.

Little opportunities, the minute particulars. They add up like loose change in a jar.

I heard the dogs scratching at the door as I walked towards the house. I opened it, and they bolted for the field. Jazz looked over her shoulder and occasionally bit Righteous on the feet trying to trip him up. Righteous ran through the field like an NFL tail back working his way through the secondary. I walked in, cranked the stereo and sat at my desk. I had some homework to do on myself. It helped me work with Bob to think back on how I had made the theoretical into the practical. In other words, how did I take the information from others and apply it to myself.

What If I Don't Like Myself?

I remember telling people early in my work that I wanted to be "myself." That was my dream. I realize now how ridiculous a statement that was. I had no real concept of who I was. Somewhere along the line I realized that if the dream was to be myself, then the first major step in preparation was to understand who I was. I realized that significant obstacles awaited me. What if I didn't like myself? What if I realized that there was nothing unique about me, nothing I really had to offer the world? If I didn't like myself, how could I possibly dream or revisit the dream of being myself?

I recently read an article about actor Mickey Rourke. As I thought back on my self-observation process, Rourke's description of his life sprang into my mind.

My life - it's 99 per cent regret right now. And that other one per cent, that's all I've got to play with. I hear people say "Mickey squandered his talent.' Well, it's more vital than that. The fact is that I squandered my life. There was a time when I knew that and I didn't care. For me it was just a way of covering up all the hurt.[6]

I resonated with two points in Rourke's confession. First was the fact that so much of what I had done to myself was to cover up the hurt, as Rourke suggested, under the illusion that somehow I was protecting myself. Second, Rourke saw that the one per cent of his life was useful. He could focus on that one percent, starting with what's right, to repair the damage.

Identifying my own process was scary. How much of my life would be regret? It was easy to think I had not achieved much in my life. I had a rocky marriage, no kids, and was back in school working on a Ph. D. My wife and I were in tremendous debt. As a college basketball player, I was a little-played reserve and a public symbol of the garbage-minutes player. The good people of Charlottesville often reminded me of that lack of success. I had sold software for five years, but I didn't exactly set the world on fire.

So what was right that I could begin with? I have been educated by, employed by, or been part of some of the best organizations in the world. I played a role on all of those teams, in all of those organizations. That was where my success resided. It was more than Rourke's one percent. It was with those successes I could start my dream process.

I had a choice to make. I either had to be content with how I was living, or I had to find a means to live in a more fulfilling way. I knew what it felt like to live the way I'd been living. It didn't feel right. No major traumas or disappointments, but a cumulative feeling of being unfulfilled. People often tell me that their lives don't feel quite right, yet they are too scared or uncertain to change. That seemed like purgatory to me. I decided to take the risk, to learn more about myself, to do the work.

As I thought back over my life, I remembered how it was to be where Bob was. It was easy to jump into the obstacles, to beat myself up over the things that were wrong. I was reminded of something interesting when I sat down with the model in front of me. I had had to fill in the dream part first. The first time I wrote out my own process I

---

[6]Jon Wild, Uncut

wrote: "To be myself." Then I moved onto preparation where I had written: "Know myself." How the hell was I going to do that? I had written: "Learn about myself." Brilliant. I was the master of the obvious. How do I learn about myself? I could go ask the people around me who they thought I was and how they experienced me. That wouldn't be enough, though, because I would merely discover and perhaps turn into who they thought I was. Much of my discomfort in life had been that so many people around me didn't know me, the real me. I needed to pay attention to how I experienced myself. Under "Learn about myself," I had written: "Pay attention."

That experience highlighted the contradiction between the statements we make about ourselves, and the observations about how we actually live. In my case, my actions created an outward aura of intimidation, of arrogance, and of acting smarter than others. While I knew those were part of me, it certainly was not the way I felt inside, nor was it the mark I wanted to leave on the world.

I had learned this cockiness on the court and in the playgrounds of downtown Washington, D. C. Cockiness was a survival mechanism. Knowledge was a weapon, my basketball skill a ticket into the dance, my confidence a projection of strength. The use of these traits to shape the world around me was a sign of my weakness. I wanted to belong; I wanted to fit in. Cocky and smart were the only ways I knew how. But it was a lie. As long as I lived that lie, I couldn't see the real me. I certainly couldn't expect others to see or to embrace the real me.

Pay Attention!

So I began to pay attention, to make observations about myself, about how other people saw me. I collected those experiences into a journal. Nothing prolific, just notes. I noticed that I always paid attention to the tough times, but I rarely processed my responses. I blamed other people for things. The blame manifested as anger. Anger seemed so powerful, especially in the world of sports. At six foot two and two hundred pounds, I could intimidate people. I learned from my friends that people hated arguing with me. That certainly was not how I wanted to live. I hated people like that. There were parts of me that I didn't like very much. Making observations required honesty, sometimes brutal, honesty. It required courage.

The good news was that anger, intimidation, needing to win were learned behaviors. My high school coach taught me to fight, to stand my ground. I rarely threw the first punch, but I never walked away either. I wasn't like that before basketball. I realized how much I liked being alone, enjoying myself, my ability to learn, to try new things, to engage in things other people might not understand. I realized that although I liked doing physical things, I could get the same feeling from intellectual pursuits as well. What I loved was the natural rhythm of learning, creating, and then expressing. That described what basketball had been for me. Then I would start over again. Under the dream, I had written: " rhythm." Under preparation I had written: "Be alone, try new things, learn."

The clock read 4 am. Going back to those first steps is always a workout. Righteous was up on the bed. Jazz waited for me to leave so she could go through the trash. I headed upstairs and climbed into bed, pulling up the cover and adjusting the pillows to cradle my recently dislocated shoulder. Man, it was hard to sleep on it. Seven knee operations, a badly broken arm, elbow surgery, dislocated and broken fingers; I knew how to deal with physical pain. The emotional traumas weren't quite as clean. No simple emotional rehab.

Righteous curled up in the bend of my knees. I kept thinking about my process. The dream was to be myself, to have my own ideas, and to express them in a responsible way. That was why teaching and counseling gave me the same feelings that playing basketball had. It was not just the physical or mental expression of something. It was the emotional creation and expression that felt so real, the emotions of the real me, whatever they were and wherever they happened. The dream was the fulfillment, the engagement between my own emotions and the world around me. It was that realization that allowed me to learn from different types of performers, from different types of people, to see beyond the physical definitions of sport and music and surgery and business. It's startling what happens when I pay attention. Through observation, I knew there was a rhythm to the way I expressed the real me.

Keeping the Desire Greater than the Fear

Bob called me two days later wanting to talk about his new life. "Man, you were right. I must have just been missing things before. I have had so much to write about. I guess I have just been so shut down I couldn't feel the bad things. I wasn't letting anything in. You really helped me, Doc."

"Don't get too excited. We still have a long way to go," I warned him.

"I know, but I have to tell you this is the best I have felt in a long time. Just seeing the little things at home and at work that feel good. Or recognizing something that makes me feel anxious, and knowing that it is the result of that experience. That has given me a sense of control I haven't had."

"Sounds good. Keep it up. I'll see you in a couple of weeks."

"So what do I do now?"

"As I said when you left, just keep observing. One thing you can look at is the process that Jeff gave you, you know, that crumpled napkin. If you listen to a song, watch a movie or see someone solve a problem at work, pay attention to how things play out. Let me know what you see. Go rent a Spielberg movie to get started, or *Jerry Maguire*. Pay attention to the plot. Then write about it to yourself."

"Gotcha. See ya." His cell phone was fading out.

Bob had called me at home. I was watching television, *Endless Summer II*, for the hundredth time. While Pat and Wingnut were flying around the world looking for the perfect wave, I had mentally mapped out what I was going to do with Bob. Specifically, a principal concern I have working with people is the two-prong task that needs to be addressed. This is the standing civil war that T. E. Lawrence described. My own experience was a prolonged battle, a war with no end. The good side of me, the parts I liked constantly skirmished with the less than desirable side.

I once heard an Olympic rower give a talk. She was asked if fear was a factor for her. She replied, "Of course, but I do whatever it takes to keep my desire greater than my fear." Drummer John Molo had said similar words to me years earlier, but I hadn't listened. Maybe I wasn't ready at that point to hear his message.

That attitude is one key to what I teach people: *keep the desire greater than the fear.*. If I focused only on the desire side, I would set the client up to, in a sense, become addicted to those things that pumped them up. If the fear isn't dealt with or diminished in some way, life is reduced to a never-ending series of motivational speeches, pumping up the desire side. In business, I hear this a lot when I give talks. The manager brings me in to rally the troops, to energize them. When I walk in for the presentation, people say "What's this month's flavor?" The chance of impacting the desire of these people is minimal.

I feel a responsibility to deal with the fears people carry with them. These fears are usually based on their past experiences. All of them are legitimate because the fear is real, so I don't negate the fear. However, if we don't deal with these fears, they will show up consistently. The challenge is timing. When is a person ready to deal with his or her fear? Will he or she work through it? In many cases, I refer people to counselors or psychologists when the fears are deep seated, and I am not trained to deal with them. Sometimes what they perceive as fear is actually worry, and worry is usually easier for me to help someone work through.

The problem of fear arises for me when we get to the point that increasing desire is not enough. At that point, my clients must make a decision about what they really want in life, because to progress they will have to do the work. Do they want to go deeper and take some risks, or are safety and not rocking the boat good enough for them? In fact, for some people this might actually be their dream. It is at this point that the questioning begins to distinguish between what they want in life and what they are actually willing to work for. Bob thinks he is doing the real work by making observations and identifying those things that feel good. In a few weeks, we will have to examine the things that get in the way of the life he wants, the way he wants his life to feel. Making observations is somewhat safe, actually dealing with what he has observed will be harder.

Chapter 3

Beyond Happiness

Wow Me!

Bob strode into my office ready to go to work. He was smartly dressed in a charcoal suit, white starched shirt, and power yellow tie.

"Looking good, Bob!" I exclaimed.

Bob stepped into the office and did a slow, yet graceless pirouette to model his sense of style.

"The wife dressed me," he laughed.

"What's the occasion?"

"I've got a big presentation today. I got my boss to agree to some of my ideas about expansion in our group. We've been hammered by the Y2K problem, but he is willing to listen to ideas beyond that. He'll have his boss there and my entire staff as well. I have 20 minutes to share my ideas and then they'll open it up for questions."

"I have an idea."

We walked down the hall to the Vice President's conference room. It looked about as close to corporate America as anything in the hospital. I figured I could help Bob get ready for his presentation as we talked. Bob was distracted as we headed towards the conference room. I could see his mind going over his presentation.

"Do you want to talk another day?"

"No. This is what I need today. I think you can help me get ready."

"Funny. That's what I was thinking."

"Great."

We walked into the conference room.

"Where will your boss be sitting?"

"Probably at the head of the table. No, his boss will sit there. He'll sit to either side of his boss."

"And where will you be?" I asked.

"Directly across from my boss."

"Okay, I'll sit here. You sit across from me." I pulled the chair away from the table and sat down, facing Bob.

I leaned back in my chair. Bob crossed his hands on the table and sat on the edge of his seat. He was already twitching nervously.

"Okay, wow me."

"What do you mean?"

"Tell me about your great ideas."

"Really? You won't know what I'm talking about."

"First of all, you're right. I probably won't, but that doesn't matter. Second, I sold computer software for five years so I can hang with the basic principles of what you're trying to accomplish."

I was allowing Bob to do a brain dump right on the table. Until he did that, we would get nowhere. He needed to purge, so I was going to let him.

Bob did his presentation. He started out slowly. He felt he was role-playing and wasn't really into it. When he saw that I was actually paying attention, he got a nervous and looked to me, **to me**, for approval. Then something magical happened: he started to focus on his ideas. He grew excited and animated. His hands left the table and joined the conversation. By the time he was finished, he was jacked.

"Bravo," I said as I applauded.

"Really? You think it was good?"

"No. I think YOU were great. I have no idea what you said. I just wanted to see if you believed what you were saying. I'd say that you do. That is the most important thing in any presentation."

"I do believe it. I just hope he does."

"You can't control that, but if you show him that you've done your homework, thought things through, and care about what you're doing, you will give yourself the best chance you have. That is all you can do. If he disagrees, listen. Look for opportunities to give him what he wants."

"Funny you should mention that. One of the things I observed this week was how I respond to him when he disagrees with me. I shut down, stop listening, and start beating myself up."

"Then what happens?"

"Nothing. I just go home and feel bad. I feel helpless. I don't want to go against him."

"Does the fact that you disagree with him mean that you can't accomplish something together?"

"No, I guess not. But it hurts when he makes me feel wrong. I feel stupid. Some of the times he is right, and then I feel even worse."

"Remember when I asked you if your boss asked you what you want, would you be able to tell him? Well, do you know what he wants?"

"I guess not. I'm not going to go ask him what he wants."

"Why not?"

"He'd think I'm being ridiculous."

"What is another way to figure out what he wants?

"I don't know."

"What have you spent the last two weeks doing?"

"Observing myself."

"And why have you been doing that?"

"To figure out what I want in my... I get it. I should observe him."

"Exactly. Observe him. Learn from him. What excites him? What does he care about?"

"That sounds hard."

"It is, but what you need to ask yourself is, 'Is it worth the effort?' "

"Why not? I'll try it. I'll start this afternoon. Instead of worrying about him disagreeing with me, I'll use it as an opportunity to learn from him and from my staff. I'll try to figure out what they want."

"Sounds good. What else happened over the past two weeks?"

"Wow. I learned a lot about myself. Where should I start?"

"Wherever you want."

"Well, I guess the most important thing I learned was that my life is not as bad as I thought."

"What makes you say that?

"There were a lot of little things that went right for me that I would normally just pass off as luck or unimportant."

"Such as?

"Well, at work, I noticed that when I dealt with my staff on a more personal level, it felt better than just getting the work done. I stopped by some of their offices to see how I could help them, instead of waiting for them to come to me with a problem. I tried to connect that experience to some of the things we talked about, you know, about ideas. I realized that if I went to them, it became my idea, and I didn't feel so put upon. I started doing that at home also.

"It just felt good to reach out to the staff, and to help them solve problems, instead of waiting for them to come to me with something. That also seemed to give us more time to deal with things, so what would normally be a fire became a project. We combined our ideas so we all had a share in the project. That felt good."

"Did that make you happy?" I asked purposefully.

"No, it was more than that. I don't know how to describe it. Yes, I do. It was fulfilling. It transcended the work or the family issues. It was more about what we wanted to accomplish. I don't know, fulfilling is the best I can come up with."

"That's fine. We'll keep trying to describe it. When I ask people how they want to feel in life, too many say happy. I don't believe that word is descriptive enough. A lot of life makes us happy or sad. But the trick is to be specific about the type of happiness you want. The people I interviewed never used the word happy to describe themselves.

They used words like fulfilled, connected, engaged in their lives. They felt there was a sense of control over the way they experienced their lives. For Jeff Rouse, he wants to feel "Easy Speed" in and out of the water. All that matters is that he knows what that feels like and what it means to him. Your task is to stay open to the feelings you're after."

"That makes sense."

Bob was still standing. The excitement he felt from his presentation stirred in him. His attention drifted between our conversation and his impending meeting with his team and bosses. When he was focused on us, he leaned forward on the table. His hands were open, palms flat, his fingers relaxed. When his mind raced to his meeting. He stood up and paced, sweaty imprints of his hands where his hands had been.

Loving to Learn

"What else did you observe?" I asked Bob.

"At home, I paid attention to how I felt when I came home from work. When things went well at work, I brought that home with me. When they didn't, I brought that home, too. One day on the way home, a song I loved in college came on the radio, and I started singing along to it. Normally, I don't really pay any attention to radio. I'm still beating myself up. When I got home that day I felt great, and I went into the kitchen singing the song and danced with my wife. That was fun. My kids came running in to see what was going on. Then they rolled their eyes and ran back upstairs. The next day I went to the record store and bought some CD's of songs I loved from college and listened to them on the way to work. Man, that made a huge difference.

"If I needed to call the office on the way in, I'd listen to the first part of the song, sing along, and then make the call. If something was going on at work, I would just ask, "How can I help?" Usually there was silence on the other end. That made me wonder how people expected me to respond. I made a commitment to myself to make it my idea to help them. If they want help, great. If not, that's fine, too."

"Sounds like you learned a lot."

"I still have a lot to learn. One thing I remembered is how much I like to learn."

"Let's keep learning then. Let's go back to good ol' Mrs. Haynes, your English teacher. How was she different than the other teachers?"

"I told you that she let me discover things about myself. She asked questions and let me correct myself. If I got something wrong, she would ask me why I had done something the way I had. Then she would look for the flaw in my thinking or what I might not know yet, but she always let me keep what I had written correctly. I guess I felt like she taught me how to learn and then let me go do it."

"Winston Churchill once said something to the effect of: 'I always like to learn, though I do not always like being taught.'"

"That's right. That's how I am. I need to discover things for myself. I like getting help, but if I am not shown the method of by which someone arrived at a certain conclusion, I don't feel as though I have really learned anything. It's not as useful as just knowing the right answer."

"Knowing how someone knows something is important because that is useful to you?"

"Right. And it feels great when I get something, when I learn something new. It feels even better when I can put it to use in a practical manner."

"You better get going. I don't want you to miss your presentation."

He looked at his watch. We had stopped with plenty of time for him to get back to his office and prepare.

He reached out his hand and said "Thanks, Doc."

"I'll see you next week. Remember the five questions I asked you. We'll talk about them next week."

He reached into his wallet and pulled out a piece of paper. "How do I want my life to feel? How will I make that happen? What gets in the way or takes it away? How do I get it back? What am I willing to work for?"

Who Had I Become?

Five simple questions. That is what life comes down to for me. I laid in bed trying to sleep, thinking back to the years of nightmares, of waking up trembling, scared, alone. My hands were under the pillow pushing it into my neck. I saw a PBS special on monkey behavior once. They showed an experiment where monkeys were separated from their mother at birth. When these monkeys slept, they bent their wrists at odd angles and pressed hard against them, hard enough to cause significant pain and wake themselves up. I knew feelings like that.

I faced away from the bed towards the near wall. Righteous was gently tucked in behind my knees and Boo rested at my feet. Sometimes it was hard for me to tell where my body ended and theirs began.

As I looked back, I could remember times when I couldn't lay in bed unless I was going to fall asleep right away. It wasn't that I had trouble sleeping, but somehow the bed became a dangerous place for me. I gave into a subconscious that was unsettled and mean. I rarely remembered the nightmares, but there was no mistaking where the feelings I woke with came from. The signs were clear: the bed torn apart, the animals sleeping across the room, the tired wrists from wrestling with the pillow, and the terrifying feeling of complete aloneness. I would welcome morning simply as an end to the torture.

Bedtime is different now. I go to bed and rest without having to sleep. I can read and listen to music and drift away slowly without fear. Mornings are a chance to live the way I want, to run towards something, not away from hobgoblins. Nighttime is merely replenishment of depleted energy. It fascinates me that the more I like my life, the more I do, the harder I exercise, the less sleep I need. I don't claim to understand it, but I don't need to. I rarely wake to an alarm clock or before the sun comes up, unless it leads to an opportunity that will also energize me. I wake when I wake, I wake when my body is ready and my heart and mind are finished sharing their hidden messages.

So what's the difference? Why has my life changed so much? Simply put, it is because I began to pay attention. I learned about myself, the good and the bad, the soothing and the terrifying, the talents and the flaws. Most of all though, I paid attention to how I wanted to feel, what feelings I would work for, and what got in their way. I committed myself to hold onto those feelings no matter what life threw at me. I did the work, and the day-to-day observations translated into useful lessons and meaningful action.

From my interviews and from my own observations of some of the people I interviewed, I noticed an important concept: life can be simple. I had made life too hard. I fought too many fights just to win, sometimes just to fight. I was seduced by the materialistic needs of others, the lure of status and acceptance. Looking back, I had lived a lie. I just hadn't paid attention to myself, to how I felt. Sometimes an occurrence like the cheers of a crowd felt good, yet always incomplete.

I wanted the fulfillment, the engagement of being in the right place at the right time doing the right thing.

My basketball career in college was an example of how I'd been seduced by external measures of success. I was a good high school player and had scholarship offers from some of the best programs in the country. Everyone around me in high school wanted me to play in the ACC, or at least at the highest level. I wanted to play on television, to go on the trips to Hawaii during Christmas, to get all the free stuff. Most of all, I wanted to feel like somebody. When we lost in the regionals in high school, I turned to another player and said, "There goes my scholarship!" What a lunkhead I was! The other guys on my team were crying their eyes out, because we hadn't played well and had lost. Most of the seniors would never play another organized game of basketball in their lives. They were losing something they truly loved. I was only concerned about a scholarship.

Who had I become? I played basketball because I loved it. It was a simple game that had room for creativity and expression. I didn't even think about getting a scholarship until my junior year of high school. But by senior year it had become foremost in my mind. As I lay in bed, the feelings of those earlier disappointments swept back over me. I thought about the times in college that I sat in the showers and cried, blaming the coaches for not playing me. I remembered trips to Hawaii, where I actually felt sorry for myself as a bench warmer, while I was running up Diamondhead. I remembered standing in a room with a teammate and a loaded gun, wishing it were over and having the means to make it happen. Why wasn't I paying attention then?

The only answer I can offer is that I had not done the mental work. I worked hard at basketball, but physically. I ran more than others, I lifted more than others, and I spent more drill time at the gym. In college, though, I did it for all the wrong reasons. No matter how much I worked at the physical part, I wasn't working on the most important parts, pure desire and overwhelming fear. Instinctively, I knew that the things I loved most were also the things that could cause the most pain. If I avoided love, then I also avoided pain. Whether it was in a relationship, or doing something I loved like basketball, I knew that loving someone or something unconditionally also meant real hurt.

I thought back about how I had thrilled to biking down a mountain at 55 miles an hour, or to performing well in a crucial game, but it had never been enough. Later, I would lie in bed, vulnerable from the day's experiences, exposing myself to the demons that lurked in the darkness.

At some level, I understood the connection, but I never honestly faced it.

I can't explain what basketball meant to me in college. I only remember how much it hurt. I turned basketball into a job. I disconnected from it emotionally. The same thing happened in my marriage. Just like Jim Skinner's father at Georgia Tech, I was working on the how, but I had lost track of why I was doing it. My sight had focused on the shiny brass ring, and I forgot to enjoy the rest of the ride. Eventually, I was just trying to hang onto the carousel, worrying too much about falling off.

Raindrops slammed against the windows of my old farmhouse, bringing me back to my own development. When I was at Bob's stage of discovery, I had learned the why of my life: that sense of rhythm. I had also learned some of the how: where the rhythm could be made to happen, who helped it, who took it away, and how to create it for myself. I had spent so many years, so many tears, waiting for someone else to create that comfortable rhythm.

By paying attention, I had learned to notice when I had the rhythm and when I didn't. I had learned to make mental notes to remind myself of both. I had invested in myself to find that rhythm. By now, each day, each hour, is about making that rhythm happen, by loving, feeling, and sharing myself with others. I had learned to listen to myself as well as others.

54

Chapter 4

Playing To Win

I Want To Be Myself

I asked Bob to meet me at Adventureland. They had batting cages and an remarkable motorcycle video game. I wanted to play some, and I knew Bob brought his kids there once in a while. Bringing the kids was different than coming with someone his own age. He probably came and watched his kids play, remembering what if felt like. I doubted that he was able to just relax and play on his own. That was why we were here today.

We sat in the parking lot, relaxed on the curb, and talked for a while. I wanted to see if he was doing his homework.

"Come up with any answers this week?" I asked.

"I'm not sure. How do I want my life to feel? That's a tough one. I mean it seems to me that we are all capable of so many different emotions and feelings. How do you choose one?"

"I'm not saying you choose one. The trick is to figure out what feels right to you in different situations. Before you came to see me, would you say that you felt all these different emotions you're talking about?"

"No. If I thought about it at all, what I felt was scared and shut down all the time. Sometimes I felt exasperated, frustrated."

"So with this wide spectrum of emotions, you were still living your life in a small range of what is possible or what is real?"

"Yeah, I guess. That never occurred to me. I guess I would've said I was too emotional. What you're saying is that I wasn't emotional enough."

"Pretty much. How about when you were a kid. How would describe your emotions then?"

"Real. Whatever I felt, I just let it out. If I was sad, I cried. If I was angry, I had a tantrum."

"How'd that feel then?"

"I don't know. I never thought about it."

"So what changed?

"I grew up. I got punished if I threw a tantrum. If I cried, my older brothers just made fun of me. That didn't feel good."

"So in a sense other people started to control your emotions. What happened if you felt really good about something?"

"When I played sports, I'd get excited and hug the guys or slap the guys on the butt. That was fun. It made me feel like I was part of something. The rest of the time, though, I was taught not to celebrate anything, to be a "good winner." I didn't really know how to be happy about something and share that with someone else. When I tried, people seemed to pull back like something was wrong with me. That didn't feel good either, so I kept my emotions to myself. Eventually I learned that if I screwed up, the best thing to do was to beat myself up publicly about it. Somehow, that was my way of showing other people that I cared. No one ever got on me for accepting blame or beating myself up. In fact, it seemed like it was expected."

"And do you still do that?"

"Sure. That gets rewarded a lot at work. I mean, if I step forward and take the blame or do something that shows I knew I screwed up and worked harder, then it is like the mistake didn't matter much. It still doesn't feel good, though."

"Basically what you're saying is that the emotions you will let show have become a way to manipulate other people to get what you want. Who controls your emotions now?"

"I think I still control them, at least how I show them to others. It still seems as if showing negative emotions is more acceptable. I know I want to be accepted, so I show those. If something good happens, I just keep it to myself. In fact, I just tuck it away and never really celebrate."

"What would you like to do?"

"When something goes well, I want to enjoy it, like Mozart enjoying his talent. I guess I just want to be myself. If I'm sad, I want to cry sometimes without being made fun of. Actually, I'd like it if I felt it was okay to cry even when I'm alone. But I always catch myself and say, "This won't do any good.""

"If I'm excited I want to be able to show it. I only do that around my kids when we're playing sports. The other night, I was helping Michael, my youngest son, with his homework. It was humbling. I saw him actually understand something for the first time about the computer. He'd been struggling with it for a long time and now he got it, because I helped him. It felt great. I wanted to hug him, but I didn't. Then he jumped out of his chair and gave this me great big hug. I just melted around him and held onto him. That's what I want to feel."

Bob's eyes softened as he imagined himself hugging his son. A sadness crept into his voice. Maybe it was love, a love of that moment and his son. I recognized it, but had never felt that. I wondered what my birth parents experience was. Did my mother have other children? Did I have brothers and sisters?

Freedom

"That kind of experience happens at work sometimes when I help somebody understand something," Bob continued. "I can see it in their eyes, but we act like we are just doing our jobs, and go onto the next project. I wish there were some acceptable way for adults to celebrate like I do with my kids, or when I play sports."

"What do you mean by acceptable?"

"I want it to be safe. I feel like I'll be judged by the people around me if I do something goofy. So I just play it safe and hold back. Actually, I think I have hardened enough so that it doesn't cross my mind to do anything but bury the feelings."

"And that feels safe?"

"I guess not, but it is predictable. It's not risky," Bob cocked his head like a quizzical puppy.

"And you don't like the way your life feels, because you're playing it safe. Yet you don't feel safe?"

"Right. Doesn't seem to add up does it?" Bob said.

"Well it adds up, but not to what you want. I hear this safety thing all the time. People tell me they want to be safe in their job, safe in relationships. Let me tell you what I think. True safety doesn't exist. Everything we do has risk. Think of everything as a cost-benefit analysis. You do those at work all the time, right?

"Of course."

"How often does your group do a cost-benefit analysis to determine if they will go forward with something?"

"On everything we do. That is how we decide. If the cost is worth the benefit, we'll take the risk."

"Right. How often do you do that with your emotions?"

"Never. At least not purposefully."

"When you do these at work, you get a pretty clear vision of the benefit of something, right?"

"Yeah." He was thinking hard. His eyes were squeezed shut as he listened. He was doing the emotional math in his head.

"So you decide where you want to be, what a product should do, what it should feel like, how it should work, what the benefit is to the customer and ultimately to company?"

"Sure. We focus on all the things we can control: the space, the hardware, and the delivery. All those things. By the time we're done, we have a good idea of what the final product should be."

"Then what do you do?"

"We start pricing things. See what we can subcontract. Look at vendors. See who we have worked with in the past and what the relationship was. If we don't like that, we seek out new vendors. Ultimately, we have a good idea of what something will cost, and how we will create the new product."

"And if the cost outweighs the benefit, do you scrap the project?"

"Of course not. We scale it back or look for alternative ways to do things."

"Right. So if I asked you to apply that process to your own life, how would you do that?"

"Geez. Who knows?"

"Well, let's start with the first question I asked. How do you want your life to feel? In a sense, you are creating a new product: you. So be creative. Forget all the limitations, all the obstacles. If you could feel anyway you want to feel, what would that be?"

"Happy."

"Not good enough. If I asked you to create a new product or service and you stopped at a product that made people happy, how would your boss respond?"

"He'd laugh or threaten my job." He laughed.

"In the same way, 'happy' is not specific enough for creating the new you. When you decide to create something new at work what usually drives it?"

"Our customers. They have a need and we try to satisfy it."

"Exactly. So what needs do you have to fulfill to make your life feel the way you want?"

"Oh. Well, freedom. I want to be free."

"Still not good enough. Define freedom for me."

"It's the lack of oppression. No limits."

"So you are now free. Nothing to worry about. No one hassling you. Here you are sitting around being free. What do you think will happen?"

"I'll get bored."

"So now do you feel free?"

"No. I'm starting to get bored and frustrated."

"When do you feel the most free?

"Playing with my kids. Sometimes with my wife. At work, it's when I know I have a project that requires some creativity. I feel the most free when I am totally absorbed in a meaningful problem that I think I will eventually solve."

"You don't worry about your boss or your job or what people will think?"

"Not until I'm driving home. But when I'm actually doing it, it feels great. I love that feeling."

"When I did my dissertation, I asked people to define freedom. Every one of them said something to the effect of not being oppressed. That was not what I expected, so I asked a different question. I went back to my friends and asked them when they felt the freest. Every one of them named some activity. I read somewhere that freedom itself is an activity. To sustain it, one cannot be passive. When I interviewed these successful people, they talked about freedom at a different level. They described a freedom of doing something, the feeling of freedom that they experienced in doing that activity. When your Dad retired he was free from work and most responsibilities, right? He didn't have to get up everyday and go to work."

"Right."

"But he didn't know what made him feel free, because he focused on the freedom *from* something. When he didn't want to be oppressed anymore. Yet he didn't know what to do to feel free."

"I see that. That makes sense to me," Bob nodded.

"So if you want to feel free, you will have to make observations about what makes you feel free. You've already named some of these things. It sounds like a sense of engagement in the things that you do makes you feel free. After you've designed a new project at work and you figure the cost, do you look internally to see what areas of the company could help you carry out the project?"

"Sure. That way we can keep the cost down, and it makes things easier in the long run. If we know a certain group in the company doesn't work well with us, we leave them out of the loop. We know from experience that paying more money to an outside vendor will be a better option in the long run."

"If you were to start looking for the feelings of freedom in your life, where would you start? You wouldn't quit your job, leave your kids and wife, or stop paying the bills, right?"

"I couldn't do that. I have too many responsibilities. Then I would feel awful. I certainly wouldn't feel free."

"Of course you wouldn't. The problem is that responsibilities smack us in the face everyday. They cry out for attention. Bills come in the mail; our boss wants to know if we've finished our work. Our wives want to know when we're coming home. Remember, though, that like responsibility, freedom takes work. It takes work to find it and hold onto it. The responsibilities don't disappear. Freedom, on the other hand, does. It slowly atrophies. It's a muscle we have to exercise. Democracy is based on the exercise of freedom by the people. Companies that rest on the past die, because the freedom of the marketplace rewards the companies that exercise the freedom to take risks."

"So how does all that relate to me?"

"I sent you to make observations about your life, to identify the places you could exercise your freedom without too great a cost. It is not always clear whether or not the consequences of freedom are worth the costs. That's true with your company, right? You don't know ho well a new product will sell, but you're willing to take the risk because you weigh the cost against the benefits."

"So how do I do that in my life?"

My first thought was that Bob had just told me he did this every day. He applied freedom and responsibility in his work, with his family and friends. The problem was that he focused too heavily on the responsibility side of the equation. He defined freedom as simply the "freedom from" perspective. He didn't need to learn responsibility. He had that down pat.

Benefit-Cost, Freedom-Responsibility

"Instead of cost-benefit, think about it as benefit-cost. It is a subtle distinction, but an important one. If you start by looking at the costs first, you kill the desire to examine the possibilities. That is why the process begins with ideas. Ideas don't demand responsibility. They can be created, then discarded. Dreams are different. They require commitment. Their demands examine benefits before costs, the dream before obstacles. You have to allow yourself to fantasize, to make believe, to hope and wonder. If we always started with the costs first, we might never progress. In fact, we are actually in a continuous, unspoken benefit-cost analysis of our lives. But even that description sounds lifeless and not very inspiring. The people I interviewed talked in livelier terms of freedoms and responsibilities. What freedoms do you want to exercise, and what responsibilities will you accept to make the freedom happen? When a bill comes in the mail, how do you feel about it?"

"Terrible. It is one more responsibility I have to face."

"The reality though is that the bill merely represents a freedom that you have already used. If it is an electric bill, you have used electricity to make your life better in many ways. Picture the guy who runs around turning off all the lights after his kids. If he does that often enough, he will end up ignoring the freedom that electricity gives him to live a certain lifestyle. He will have forgotten the freedom and see only the cost. But we all make a decision every month that says the cost of electricity outweighs the cost of not having it. How about your job? You get paid, and sometimes you actually like the things you do. Yet you moan about your job all the time instead of really appreciating the freedom it gives you."

"That all makes sense, but everyone does that. I don't think I'll be changing that anytime soon."

"I'm not asking you to. What I'm suggesting is that you need to do some real soul searching when answering the question: 'How do I want my life to feel?' Are there things in your life in which the freedoms so outweigh the responsibilities that when you do them, the freedom feels breathtaking and permeates the rest of your life?"

"I don't know. I'll have to think about that."

"Exactly. And you'll have to keep thinking about it for the rest of your life. When you were a kid, the sense of play you had carried over into all kinds of things. You were curious about everything. Then responsibilities crept in, you did your chores and homework, went to school, right? But when you played, you played. You engaged in the games, in learning new things, in putting a new carburetor in the car. When you worked on weekends to make extra cash, you knew you were doing it so you could fix the car or have enough money to go out with someone. That made it worth it, right?"

"Of course. It didn't make work fun, though. I would rather have been playing."

"Sure, but, still, the sense of play was how you described those days. As we grow older, we become less dependent on other people to provide for our basic needs. We start caring for ourselves. Day by bay, our sense of play gives way to covering our basic needs. That can be overwhelming. By definition, we become more responsible for our circumstances, but we only accept that so we can maintain our freedom. As that happens, the things we didn't worry about as kids become more burdensome, because our focus must shift to "freedom from": freedom from the elements, freedom from hunger, freedom from poverty. When we get our first house or our first job or our first car, it feels great. Pretty soon, though, those things that felt free turn into sources of responsibility. That happens because we spend so much time fulfilling the responsibility, we lose sight of the freedom to do things or the experience of freedom when we do them. They seem less important, trivial sometimes. We lose our sense of play, of being engaged in our own lives."

"So what do I do about it?"

"You've already started by trying to figure out how you want your life to feel. For Jeff Rouse, it was that sense of Easy Speed. You are trying out feelings of freedom. It might change as you make more observations. For now, focus on that. Where and when and with whom in your life do you feel free? Remember that napkin Jeff gave you?"

Bob pulled it out of his pocket. "I carry it with me all the time." There were more notes on it. It was a mess.

"The next step then is Preparation. In other words, how do you make those feelings happen? Part of preparation is the freedom-responsibility or benefit-cost analysis. In truth, the freedom-responsibility relationship drives the whole process. In coming to me, in having new ideas and trying to figure out your dream or how you want life to feel, you've already used it. The cost of not doing something about your life was too high for you. You decided to exercise your freedom by coming to me and engaging in this process. You exercised your freedom by making observations about yourself. People who don't exercise their freedom just make statements about themselves from the experiences of years ago. In preparation, you are going to specifically map out the things that give you a sense of freedom. You're going to weigh the cost, and you're going to look for alternative sources of those feelings."

"I talked to a couple of friends of mine, and they said going after the feelings you want is like being an addict. Why wouldn't someone just take drugs or drink or be completely irresponsible?"

"Because the cost is too high. Every action you take will have consequences. Most people care about the people around them, and they don't want to do anything to hurt them. If people came to me that didn't care about the people around them, I'd send them to a therapist. But the people I interviewed and most of the people I work with know that if they hurt someone else, the ultimate consequence will be the loss of the free feelings. There is always a balance. Usually people who do those things are convinced that what happens to others who take unnecessary risks won't happen to them. No one takes drugs hoping they will become a drug addict, or even thinking it will happen to them. Those people just don't consider the realities when they make choices. We're talking about real life here.

"The key is figuring out what is really important in life, and accepting the responsibilities that relate to your chosen freedoms. If someone else wants you to do something for him or her on a consistent basis, you'll have to get something in return. That sounds selfish, but it isn't. I do this work all the time, and I get something each time I do it. Why do you think I haven't charged you yet? I love the one-on-one of helping. It makes me feel free. Whenever I decide to do it as my principal source of income, I'll have to charge people for my time, so I won't have to worry about the other responsibilities. I haven't asked you for a thing yet, right?"

"I was wondering when that would happen."

"The truth is that currently I meet most of my relatively modest needs from other sources, and the satisfaction from you is that you'll do the work. Just by being you, working at this the way you are, you are giving me something. Do you think I am being selfish?"

"No, just the opposite."

"One of my best friends is a professional drummer, John Molo. I've known him since high school. One of the coolest, nicest people I have ever met. He plays a hundred shows in some years. Travels. Stays in lousy towns. He is often alone in the hotel. He is away from the family the loves. I asked him once how he keeps from burning out. He told me that he never confuses what he gets paid for with what he loves to do. He plays the drums for free. He gets paid for the travel, the time away from his family, the loneliness. He only gets to play drums a few hours a day, but he has decided that benefit of getting to play the drums far outweighs the cost.

"At one time in his life, he thought about quitting. He was tired of the life. He was going to be a salesman. His wife grabbed him and told him that he needed to wake up. She knew him well enough to know that he would hate being a salesman, and that the cost would be too great. She reminded him of the benefit side of playing the drums, because he had focused on the cost side.

"Molo has also realized that when he plays the drums, the performance of the whole band depends on him. He sets the tempo for the group. Part of the experience for John is how well he interacts with the people around him. In fact, both Bruce Hornsby, the pianist, and Molo are described by the people they play with as making them better. In fulfilling their own life, they make other people better. I don't run into many people who don't want to feel that way."

"My head is beginning to hurt." Bob rubbed his temples. "This is a lot to digest."

I stood up and started swinging the bat. "That's why I wanted to meet here. It'll make sense to you after we play a while."

I poked his gut with the end of the bat. He grabbed it and wrestled it from my hands. He took a slow swing at me and I bolted.

"Motorcycles first. I'm going to kick your ass!" I exclaimed.

Dawn Staley Meet Hans-Georg Gadamer

I loved the motorcycle game because it had a real-life feel to it. You leaned into turns and used your weight and rhythm to control the bike. You could also compete side-by-side with someone. Bob pulled out a $20 bill and fed it into the machine. Looked like we were going to be here a while. He grabbed the tokens and we headed to the motorcycles. There were two kids on them and I could see the disappointment on Bob's face. He was ready, impatient. I tried to enjoy the kids having fun, talking smack to each other, and getting excited when they wrecked. They didn't have extra tokens lined up to the side so I figured this was their last ride. Their race came down to the wire with the smaller of the two kids crouched down low trying to be more aerodynamic (not that it really mattered on a video game). The smaller kid won, but they high-fived each other as they dismounted.

"Let's go do the snowboard game!" said the bigger kid.

"Cool!" replied the littler one as they sprinted across the room.

I turned back to the motorcycles and saw Bob already mounted on the left side. "I like this side better."

"Whatever."

We stayed on the motorcycle game until my butt was sore. Bob wanted to keep going. So far we were about even in victories. I'd lost count of how many times we played. I was having fun watching Bob. As soon as the coins dropped in he was all business. I fell into deeper thought.

Bob reminded me once again of the philosopher, Gadamer, who talked about play. Gadamer argued that, "First and foremost, play is self presentation." That was the essence of what I had heard from the people I interviewed, that they were most themselves when they played, so they made their lives about play. Gadamer went on to say:

Play fulfills its purpose only if the player loses himself in the play: seriousness is not merely something that calls us away from play; rather seriousness in playing is necessary to make play wholly play. Someone who doesn't take the play seriously is a spoilsport. [7]

Bob was serious about this game.

I had interviewed Dawn Staley, one of the best women basketball players in this country during the late nineties. A two-time National Player of the Year in college, Dawn provided the best description of performance I had ever heard. In fact when I showed others, such as pro football all-star Howie Long and Surgeon Curt Tribble, what Dawn said they both said "Exactly right! That is why I do what I do."

Dawn was a difficult interview. She is bright, but very quiet. She eventually grew exasperated with my questions. She was trying out for the Olympic team in 1996 soon after I interviewed her. She slammed her fist down on the table and said:

Winning the gold medal is my goal, not my dream. My dream is about playing to win as often as possible with and against the best women basketball players in the world. Winning the gold medal as a goal gives me some direction, but my dream is something I need to live everyday. And I'm doing that each time I play to win. ...When I'm playing to win, that's when I feel resonance. If I win, that's great. I want to win and having the gold medal as my goal forces me to play to win. But what I love to do, what my dream is, is to play to win.

Dawn had captured Gadamer's idea exactly. Now many people would have read that and thought she was talking about winning. Sure

---

[7] Hans-Georg Gademer, Truth and Method (New York: The Continuum Publishing Company, 1994).

she wants to win, but if that were all she cared about, she would play against people she knew she could beat. She wanted to play against the best, because the demands of that experience forced her to use all of her capabilities, all of herself, to pursue her goals. In Gadamer's words playing to win transcends sport and becomes about life:

The self-presentation of human play depends on the player's conduct being tied to these make-believe goals of the game, but the meaning of these goals does not in fact depend on their being achieved. Rather in spending one's self on the task of the game, one is in fact playing oneself out.[8]

Dawn Staley, street kid from Philly, meet Hans-Georg Gadamer, world famous philosopher. Dawn had taken Gadamer once step further. She said that being engaged, living the dream, also gave her the best chance to perform well and achieve. This theme was consistent in the lives of the interviewees.

Bob and I were exhausted, but energized. Bob wanted to keep going. He was having a blast. I had won the last race, which led to him buying my soda. He wanted redemption. Bob was holding the bat now, ready to hit the batting cages. This was a teachable moment I needed to take advantage of.

"So what did you learn from that."

"That I need to lean more on the right hand turns," he chuckled, " I know, I know, that's not what you meant. Well, let's see."

"Did some of the races feel better than the others?"

"Yeah. I caught myself worrying more about where you were sometimes, than what I was doing."

"And why do you think that happened?"

"I wanted to win. I love to win."

"But what happened when you focused on winning?"

"I lost."

"What happened in the races that you won?"

---

[8] Ibid

"I was more focused on what I felt like. Using your word, I was more engaged in the race, in driving the motorcycle. I was completely focused. It didn't feel like I was trying as hard, but I was doing better."

"Easy Speed?"

"Yeah. Easy Speed."

I told him what Dawn had shared with me.

"How does that apply to what we just did?"

"I knew I wanted to win, but I was having more fun just racing. I see where you're headed. By being engaged in the race, I was also racing better."

"Right. And how did that feel when you were totally engaged and you won?"

"It felt great. I wanted to do it again. I was energized."

He was jacked as he talked. The bat in his hands was flying all over the place. He sent my soda flying across the room. "Sorry," he murmured. I expected him to be embarrassed, but he just kept talking as he walked over to get me a new soda.

Performance By Design

Bob walked back towards me, almost spilling my new soda as he thrust it into my face. He remained standing, pacing around the table. My neck tired as I watched.

"But how do I apply that to my life," Bob asked. "I mean I can't ride motorcycles all day. I have other responsibilities. I think I would get tired of riding these damn things all day anyway."

"We'll get there. I'll explain the concept a little better, but remember the process? The whole point is that these feelings can happen in everyday life in places you might not realize. The process is a structure that helps you create more opportunities for those feelings.

"Remember Molo, the drummer. He can't play the drums all day either. He has to travel, set up, deal with record companies. He has many of the same responsibilities you have. But he knows he can get those feelings, that he can engage himself when plays the drums. He also knows he has to seek those opportunities out. He needs to protect them. Playing the drums gives him energy that allows him to get through the tasks that drain energy. His responsibilities are directly related to the feelings he wants to have everyday. That makes them worth doing. It gives responsibility a purpose. Benefit-cost. Freedom-responsibility."

"So by making observations about myself, about my life, I can see the things that may already give me those feelings?"

"Exactly. It's like your company creating a new product. Once you know what the product will look like, you look internally to see how the other parts of the company can help you build it. Too often people think that to have the feelings we're talking about, they need to go outside of the life they have already created. My experience is that these moments happen in most people's lives, but they happen by accident. Remember Rouse said that many of his races happened by accident, that Easy Speed happened by accident?"

Bob thought for a minute closing his eyes and lowering his head.

"Yeah, then he said that the process made him realize that he could train for Easy Speed, that he could design his performance."

"But he also acknowledged that he couldn't make it happen all the time," I reminded Bob. "He acknowledged that he couldn't control winning. He focused on making Easy Speed happen when he could, because through observation he knew it energized him, felt great, and that he performed best when he achieved Easy Speed. He went to work learning how to make Easy Speed happen, what took it away or kept it from happening, and then on getting it back. The process."

"Jeff also said he feels he could make that happen in every part of his life," Bob said. "He believes that even without a special talent like swimming, he could find the equivalent of Easy Speed in his life. That is what you're trying to teach me."

"That is what you're learning. I can't teach you what you can't learn. I'm just telling you how to find it. You are the only one that can find it for yourself. The process depends on your participation, because you are the only factor you have control over. I could never have come up with Easy Speed for Jeff. I work with doctors, but I know little about medicine. What I'm showing you is *how* people know what they know, not *what* they know. It's up to you to apply it."

"Got it. It's not easy though."

"I never said it was easy. In fact, it is hard to do consistently. I struggle with it at times. The question is whether or not having this lifestyle is worth it, comparing between freedom and responsibility or benefit and cost. You already know that for you, the cost of the conflict is too high. You do not accept having the feeling of responsibility outweigh the feeling of freedom. That probably has some impact on how well you actually perform your responsibilities. The cool part is that there are times when you can feel free **and** fulfill your responsibilities.

"That is what the people I interviewed talked about. Combining the two whenever possible. In Molo's case, the record or the booking company executives certainly don't say to themselves, "Let's pay John Molo to fly all over the country and be away from his family." They are paying him to play the drums. But he decides the relationship between freedom and responsibilities for himself. When he plays the drums, he gets a paycheck.

"In your case, you love to solve problems, to create, to work as part of a team. There is a sense of freedom in that for you. Then there are times at work that are pure responsibility. What you need to observe is whether or not you can create a healthy balance between the two in your current situation. That takes homework and thought. Is it worth it to you to find that out? Is it worth the work to protect what you create? I can't answer that for you."

"I can't answer that yet, either. But I am curious. I want to try."

"That's all you can do. Let's go hit."

We headed to the cages and hit balls for a while. I loved the feeling of the bat in my hand, the soft crack of the bat, the line drive up the middle. Bob was struggling a bit next to me. He hadn't done this in a while. Slowly he loosened up and was hitting his own line drives. I stopped and watched him hit for a while. He didn't notice I was watching. I told him to keep his head on the ball. I deliberately screwed him up. He kept missing the ball, fouling it back. He turned and glared at me.

"Don't think I don't know what you're doing," he scowled.

"Then fix it." I laughed and took a few more swings. Bob asked if he could use the 20-year-old Pete Rose bat I was using. "Sure." I hoped he wouldn't break it.

Soon enough, I heard the sweet sound of wood on ball, and the not so sweet sound of Bob grunting. He looked back at me and smiled. He was learning again what he'd known before. The question for him, for everybody, is can they trust what they know?

Learning To Fly

I left that night to fly to Los Angeles to do some interviews. Sitting in the airport, I heard over the loudspeaker that a flight to Cincinnati had been delayed for a couple of hours. A collective groan echoed throughout the terminal as people slammed books shut and sprinted to the phones. Most of the anger came from white males in suits that had been purchased years earlier when they were still in shape. I turned up the volume on my Walkman and went back to my book. Several minutes later, a little boy crashed into my feet. He looked up at me with a huge smile on his face as his father came rushing over and apologized. I smiled and said, "No problem."

I watched them walk back to an empty space, the father brushing dust off the boy's pants. Then they did something remarkable. While other parents were stuffing food and books into their children's hands, this father and son were playing. The little boy got into a batter's stance, his hands around an imaginary bat. His father helped him position his hands and feet and then walked about twenty feet away. "Bottom of the ninth, two out and Mark McGuire steps to the plate. The Cards are down one, a man on first. Mcguire has one home run already today. The crowd is on its feet."

The father was doing the play by play as he went into the pitching motion with nothing in his hand. He wound up and released: nothing! The little boy swung as hard as he could. He stood at the imaginary plate and watched the ball sail far over the father's head. The father faded back slowly looking at the ceiling, his hands up over his head as if he were going to catch something. Then he stepped hard into the wall and dropped his head as if the ball had cleared the stands. The little boy lifted his arms and did a slow trot around the bases, high-fiving the base coaches. "Let's play again, Dad!"

I smiled at the times my dad and I had played ball in the yard. I remembered the stories he told of playing stickball in the streets of depression-riddled New York City. Some middle-aged guy in a suit stepped on my foot and brought me back to the angst-ridden airport. The father and son continued their game. I pulled out my camera and took some pictures to keep the moment and, more important, the lesson.

What made these two different from all the others in the airport? One idea stuck in my mind. *Freedom is an activity*. It does not just happen and it is not without cost. Several people in the airport rushed by the kid and his dad making disparaging remarks. The father and son just kept playing. They weren't going to give their freedom away. They were going to exercise the freedom they had. They certainly seemed happier than others in the airport. I was certainly enjoying watching them. As I rose to board my plane, I walked over to them and simply said, "Thanks." The father smiled understandingly. As I walked away, the little boy asked, "Daddy, what did that man want?"

On board, I stood patiently as several people wrestled with their oversized packages. Whenever I fly, I am reminded of a quote from Charles Lindbergh. He once said that, "Building an airplane is easier than the evolutionary process of the flight of a bird. I'd rather be around birds." How true! Watching a bird fly is certainly more inspiring than being on a winged bus crammed with people eating bad food at thirty thousand feet. I'm sure the naval pilots I talked with on the U.S.S Eisenhower have a different experience. Most of us, though, treat flying as a necessary evil to escape the world behind us.

Flying also made me think about the relationship between freedom and responsibility. These people were just being selfish carrying oversized luggage aboard. It slowed things down and made the flight attendants' jobs much harder. Airplanes are a great study in behavior. I bet I could choose which people I wanted in my life, simply by watching how they acted on airplanes.

One thing I noticed about myself on airplanes occurs when the plane lands. As soon as the little bell dings telling the attendants that we can begin to disembark, most of the people in the plane stand up and start reaching for the overhead bins. People near the windows stand in this uncomfortable bent over position leaning on the seat in front of them.

I used to do that too. I was always impatient and felt stress flowing through me. Stress then turned into anger, as I grew more impatient. One day I was reading a book I really liked and stayed seated until the flight attendant asked me whether I was getting off or not. What I focused on was how much better it felt. Now I just sit on planes until everyone else has disembarked, and take my time getting off. It is one of the simple things that have helped me feel the way I want to. Observation turned into preparation.

I settled into my seat, pulled out my Walkman and dove into my book. The flight attendants went into their version of a pre-game talk. They held up the little margarine tub with plastic attached, this high-tech life-saving device that seemed more likely to muffle our screams when we plummet to earth than anything else. A good friend of mine once pointed out that the flight attendants had a good message for life: "Put your oxygen mask on first before assisting someone else with theirs." A simple message, but right on the mark. The best way to be able to help someone else is to help yourself first.

When I first went back to graduate school, I wanted to help people avoid the same mistakes I had made as an athlete and as a person. Several years into the program, though, I had done the book learning, but realized I still wasn't any better off than before. I started working on myself, and people started telling me how much I was changing. They wanted to know how I had done it. The difficulty is that they wanted a step-by-step, cookbook list of the things I had done.

I still run into this with people who want me to do the work for them. Eventually, what I learned about teaching the process to others was to ask the five basic questions and then make observations. For each of us, this meant risking that we won't like all of what we see. It meant looking back on our lives and understanding why we did some of things we did. This is risky for many people including me.

It also means challenging the beliefs that people close to you instilled in you as you grew up. That is always difficult for people to do, because it feels disrespectful. What made me willing to look, to take that risk? I can only guess that I just felt frustrated and angry enough about my life to take the risk. I was also confident that I could do something about it. I had some control over my own life. Blaming other people never seemed to get me anywhere. Again I just paid attention. By paying attention, dealing with my emotions without letting them swerve me into a safer life, I was able to take responsibility for my own actions and my own desires.

That sense of responsibility gave me a measure of control over my life. The more I increased my freedom from my own bad habits and poisoned beliefs, the more I could accept responsibility. The more relevant responsibility I took on and lived up to, the more freedom I gained. Knowing I wanted to feel different about myself and about my life made it easier to figure out what I wanted to feel. I began to gain some direction and momentum in that direction. Suddenly, I started learning from everything and everybody.

I am a lot better now at helping people who want to discover the life that is within them and around them. It means letting go of old beliefs and paying attention to the mess we get ourselves into. We all do it. I still do it. I have yet to meet the person who is entirely free of it. But I have enough experience to know that I will eventually get out of the mess, and that I will survive the hurt that it causes me.

It troubles me that I haven't any answer for how to help people who are paralyzed by fear, and who defend a life they don't really believe in.

Fortunately, most people I work with will only defend themselves for a time, until they start listening to their own arguments and hear how ridiculous they sound. They will defend their existing lives and values, until they start to pay attention to their feelings and what led to those feelings. The process begins to work only when they start with the dream and stop skipping right to obstacles. This is difficult, because so many things remind each of us everyday about our cares and responsibilities. Rarely does something come into our awareness reminding us of the small things in our lives that add up to real happiness. We have to give ourselves the freedom to create our own process that reminds of those special moments on a regular basis. No one else will do that for us.

Social Acceptability

The movie on the flight that day was: "Phenomenon." I loved that movie, because it was a hyperbolized representation of the process. It's about a fellow who has the special ability to have an incredible number of ideas, and then to make most of them happen. John Travolta plays George Malley, an auto mechanic who is loved by everyone in his small town. All of a sudden he is brilliant. He is no longer perceived to be the George Malley everyone else knew. They are frightened by his newfound brilliance. He feels ostracized and frustrated. He wants everyone to understand, but he doesn't know how to make that happen.

In the work I do, many people ask me about the social acceptability of going after the life you want. It is a good question. I always respond with a question: "What do you mean by socially acceptable?" It is not a quibble. What is socially acceptable in one setting might not be accepted somewhere else. When I give talks to college students, I hear many of them say that they are choosing a career to satisfy what their parents' want for them. After all, their parents paid for college. I got an athletic scholarship, and my parents were happy that I went to college at all, given the little academic work I had done in high school.

Responding to their parents' dreams, rather than their own, does pose a difficult dilemma for many of these students. For John Molo, becoming a professional musician was not socially acceptable in the town where he grew up. When he finished high school, he went to the University of Miami, which had a great music program. He surrounded himself with people who believed in what he was doing and would challenge him and teach him what it really meant attempting to be a musician. He met Bruce Hornsby at Miami and they clicked and played together for more than twenty years. When John came back for his 20-year high school reunion, he ran into someone who didn't quite understand:

I went to my high school reunion. I'm walking next to this woman, and she asks me what I do for a living. I told her I'm still playing drums. She goes, "Oh!" like she feels sorry for me. This is classic. She asks me, "Are you able to make a living?" Man that was one of the best I ever heard. Like: "Don't you have another job?" I said, "No, that's it." Later somebody came up to me while she was standing there and said, "That's John Molo. He plays on MTV." That was great.

That's one of the differences about living in L.A. I walk up to someone and say I play the drums and they say, "Great. With who?" Out East It's like: "You play drums? Oh, that's too bad. What do you really do for a living?" I guess it does sound funny. I just sit down behind those things and play.

The question each of us needs to ask is: what is the cost of doing what is socially unacceptable or socially marginal? Anything illegal clearly crosses a line that has severe consequences that will limit freedom. But in addition to the legal considerations of an action, there are the consequences of our actions on those around us. Lawrence's standing civil war surfaces again. How do we choose between doing what feels right inside of us, and doing what people around us expect of us?

My experience is that you can only answer that question by doing the work such as testing ideas, getting feedback, and analyzing what happened. What are the benefits of going after what you want and who you are? Is the cost of taking action really greater than denying yourself, simply for the acceptance of others? What do you have to give up from your present and past to have what you want in the future? Sadly, too many people answer this question without really thinking it through. Alexis de Tocqueville wondered about the cost of social acceptability when he visited America. In is defining work *Democracy in America* he wrote that:

The authority of a king is physical, and controls the actions of men without subduing their will. But the majority possesses a power that is physical and moral at the same time, which acts upon the will as much as upon the actions, and represses not only all contest, but all controversy. I know of no country in which there is so little independence of mind and real freedom of discussion as in America....

Under the absolute sway of one man, the body was attacked in order to subdue the soul, but the soul escaped the blows that were directed against it and rose proudly superior. Such is not the course by tyranny in the democratic republics; there the body is left free, and the soul enslaved. The master no longer says, 'You shall think as I do or you will die,' but he says, 'You are free to think differently from me and to retain your life, your property, and all that you possess; but you are henceforth a stranger among your people.' [9]

I think de Tocqueville underestimated the average American's independence of mind, but he put his finger on an important force, the fear of being "a stranger among your people."

The fear of not fitting in, of being ostracized, diminishes the ability of so many to take risks and to explore themselves, that their focus turns outward. People are paralyzed by the impending sense of loss rather than the hope of what they might gain. Too many people think that it is an all or nothing proposition.

The idea is to take small steps. Test something to see if it is what you want or if your perceptions are accurate for what something will feel like. Are the resulting consequences what you expected? I started by learning how people I wanted to live like actually created their lifestyles. I paid attention to the feelings I had around those people. The information I gained from them was invaluable towards weighing the benefit against the cost. Increased freedom always comes with increased responsibility. I was able to avoid some of the mistakes that others made, because they had experienced them and could talk about them.

---

[9] Alexis de Tocqueville, De la Democratie en Amerique (On Democracy in America) (New York: Plenum Press).

The plane landed at LAX, and as expected the people around me jumped to their feet. We were delayed for a while waiting for them to open the door. People grew impatient. It struck me that the many of the older people on the plane merely sat with smiles on their face. Finally, the line of people started to move. One guy yelled "Moooo!" as they were herded into the terminal. I walked out to the baggage carousel, and sure enough the luggage hadn't come out yet. The phones were jammed with my fellow passengers, as the suits paced off their nervous energy. I knew what Lindbergh was talking about. I'd rather be around birds, too.

Chapter 5

Success?

I was living The American Dream… and not my own.

-Phil Gordon
Professional Poker Player

To be totally engaged with all my functions, all my faculties, all my capacities in life. To me, that would be success.[10]

-Jacob Needleman,
"Money and the Meaning of Life"

The American Dream

I met Bob at Sloan's, a local restaurant. This was his turf. He had invited me into his life. He introduced me to several of his colleagues. My guess was that he had been telling them about the work we were doing. I knew they had questions. People learn the process at a tacit level first and then gain control over it as they articulate it. When others ask questions that they cannot articulate answers to, doubt begins to creep in. I knew this had happened to Bob. It happens to everyone. Actually this is where they can learn the most. It is easy to pump people up, to get them excited in a relatively safe place.

The challenge is to stand firm at the most crucial moments, when the fear is the greatest. That is when the potential benefit, the feelings of the most intense freedom are the greatest. As a result, the perceived cost is higher. The cost is not of losing something you have. The cost is in the loss of hope, or the realization that everything you've worked for might be lost. It is in those times, ironically, that feeling the way you want is the most important.

I shook hands with Bob's three co-workers. Lisa was a VP of customer service. She was in good physical shape, and looked younger than she probably was. She took good care of herself. Andy was a member of Bob's staff. He was puffing away on an unfiltered Camel. He was clearly out of shape and had gray skin. He looked like a blue-collar guy in a white-collar world. Mark was an executive VP. He was smartly dressed with his starched shirt and Hugo Boss suit. I could tell

---

[10] Jacob Needleman, Money and the Meaning of Life (New York: Doubleday Books, 1994)

he had questions. I ordered a draught Bass and bellied up. Bob looked a little flustered. I had a sense he was looking to me to rescue him. A little knowledge can be a dangerous thing when coupled with enthusiasm.

As I expected, Mark dove right in. He wondered about the dream-goal relationship and suggested what I was teaching was irresponsible.

"Isn't the good old American Dream to have a house, two cars, and 2.4 kids? Or to become a millionaire? Those sound tangible to me." I'd been through this many times and used thousands of bar napkins to make my points. I grabbed another napkin and pretended to doodle on it. Unbeknownst to them, I was drawing The American Goal, the path to success as it had been recited to me hundreds of times from unfulfilled people.

Success

Have kids

Borrow the money to buy a house

Get married

Borrow the money to buy a car

Get a good job

Go to a good college

Get good grades in school

"Sure, but that dream was conceived at a time when our country was developing. The goals of a society, though, change over time. Why do you think so many people wanted the house, the car, the million dollars?"

"To be successful."

"And do you have all those things?"

"Well, not the million dollars." They were all nodding.

"Do you feel successful?" I paused as they looked at my chart of goals on the napkin. I wanted it to sink in.

"You all thought by completing or achieving this list of goals, you would feel successful. So why don't you feel successful?" I asked and paused again.

Lisa spoke up. "I feel like at any moment, I could lose everything. If the stock price of our company drops too low, I'm out of a job."

"So how does that affect the way you relate to your family?"

Mark joined in. "I worry for them. I worry that I can't sustain the standard of living I've created for them."

Andy nodded. He pulled his cigarettes out of his pocket and pounded the pack against his open palm. I always wondered why smokers did that. I made a note to ask him later.

"And if you do get the million dollars, what will happen then?"

"Same thing. We'll just raise our standard of living to meet our income."

"So the treadmill never stops?"

"I guess not," Lisa whispered.

Andy joined in. "I thought this guy made you feel better about yourself," he said to Bob.

Resonance

Bob laughed. He wanted to tell Andy to slow down, to not jump ahead. I'm sure he remembered me telling him the same thing.

"That's okay," I told them. "I'm answering your questions, but you are asking me the wrong questions. You're asking me about the things that are wrong. You are looking for the faults in my logic, rather than understanding it first."

Bob jumped in with a smile. "Benefit-cost, not cost-benefit."

"Right. Instead of challenging me on the dream-goal distinction, try it out first. Think about yourself. I don't care if you accept it. The question is what's right for each of you? That's for you to decide. If you're interested in what I do, doesn't it make sense to understand the concept first, rather than attack it? I'm not going to argue that it's perfect. But from my work it seems to be a useful way for people to look at their own lives. Once you understand it better, I'd be glad to argue with you anytime, anywhere. I love that."

"Well, I think I understand it at some level, and Mark asked me something I couldn't answer," Bob said. He seemed to trust me enough now to challenge me.

"Shoot."

"Ask him yourself Mark."

Mark stopped leaning on the bar, put his beer down and looked me dead in the eyes. My guess was that he felt he had me simply because Bob hadn't been able to answer the question.

"I read a great book called Flow by some guy with a difficult name."

"Mihalyi Csikszentmihalyi. He goes by Mike. I've met him."

Mark seemed less confident. "Athletes talk about the thing they call the zone. Mike called it flow. It sounds cool and I have actually felt these things before. It sounds to me like you've just renamed those things."

"Maybe. How would you describe the zone or flow?"

"The term I would use is optimal performance. Things are effortless; time flies by; it's productive. It feels great. I'm jacked."

"How many times in your life have you actually felt that?"

Lisa jumped in. "Not many, but I know the feeling."

"Have you heard of anyone being able to achieve the zone on a regular basis?"

"Not even Michael Jordan did that."

"Right. So in doing my research, I found that these high level performers understood that the zone is a difficult goal to achieve. They knew that real life has its ups and downs. But even when they weren't in the zone, they still had pleasurable experiences that might have had some hurt in them, but the benefit usually outweighed the cost. Bob, when you met Jeff Rouse, what did you think he would be like?"

"I thought he would be really intense, have a lot of energy."

"And?"

"And he was really laid back. Not what I expected. He was a regular guy."

"The performers I talked with were not the kind that go around high-fiving people. There is a low buzz about their lives like a power line that continuously has juice going through it. They might sometimes achieve the zone, but they knew it was difficult to predict or control. So the decision they made about their lives was that they want to have this continuous flow of energy. They want to feel it, use it, be able to create it and protect it."

"That makes sense," Lisa said.

"I also thought the zone was where we should live, but given what we know today, that seems like a pipe dream. I wanted a more practical, useful view of life. When I started showing others what I'd learned, I was surprised to hear how they experienced it. People reported back that they didn't have as many bad days as they used to and that their bad days weren't as bad they used to be. I thought that was a pretty good result. They also reported more experiences with the zone. Not many, but enough that it made me realize that they were allowing the zone to happen by having fewer bad days.

"What I am after in my life, what I share with others that I learned from these performers is that being engaged in my life is what mattered. Knowing what matters to me, experiencing what matters, being myself. That took a lot of work. It meant making some meaning out of the past, being in the present, and working for the future. That isn't always going to be a high. Some days it is a struggle, but it seemed worth it to me. I realized that when I can be myself, then I can give my full attention to the task at hand, whatever it is. The more meaningful the work, the more I engage, the better results I produce."

"What's all that got to with flow or the zone," quizzed Mark.

"The point is that being engaged can happen at different levels. If you believe that the zone is the ultimate goal, then when you're not in it, not being in it will distract you. If we knew how to create it, then that would be okay. We would just work to be there. Same thing with flow. If we understood how to create it, then that would be useful. If you know people who can teach you to get you there, go talk to them. I just don't know anyone like that. Even in Mike's work, he suggests that it is difficult to achieve.

"What I learned was how to be engaged in my life more often than not, enough to be useful and make a difference. That is what the process is all about. And if one day you wake up and are disengaged, there are concrete steps you can take to re-engage. It might take a day or so, but it can be done. What I help people do is identify for themselves how to re-engage. Some days that engagement will be in flow, some days it will be in the zone. Other days, the engagement will be a struggle, but the experience will still feel better overall, than if you were not engaged at all.

"I call that sense of engagement resonance. It is a seamless fit between the person you are inside: your ideas, your goals, your talents, your faults, and the environment you are interacting with: where you are, whom you are with, the things you are doing. You are doing the right thing for the right reasons at the right time. My belief is that the experience of that is what people really desire. The benefit outweighs the cost." I turned our attention back to the napkin with the goals on it.

"What I am saying it is not the achievement of these goals that creates that feel or satisfaction or fulfillment. It is choosing goals that help you feel the way you want to feel as you pursue them AND choosing the specific goals that when reached heighten how you feel. Most people I know have these goals and most of them have achieved them or will achieve them.

"One of the guys I interviewed was a part of a startup software company that was eventually bought by Cisco for ninety-five million dollars. He accepted a big bonus to stay on board at Cisco. After a few months he went on vacation in Bali and came back and quit his job. He summed it all up by saying "I was living the American Dream... and not my own." He had achieved these goals, but was unhappy. He was happier being involved in the startup, creating the company, locking himself away for hours and working at his computer. He became a professional poker player and toured the country in an RV and raised money for cancer research. What does that tell you?"

"These are the wrong goals?" Andy said sheepishly as he pointed to the napkin.

"No, that they're insufficient or not specific enough. These goals are not about how you want to feel. In fact, they're not about you! They're simply guidelines, milestones even. Most of all, I think this is a minimum, a safety net for people who don't have a dream. Maybe they are a way for us to say we've been responsible in our lives. There is simply not enough information in this list of goals. You have to fill in the rest. What school do you want to go to? What career would you like to have? What kind of car engages you, but is affordable? What would make a happy marriage? You have to answer those questions for yourself."

"How do we do that?" Andy asked as he sat forward, suddenly more interested.

"By paying attention to how you feel, how you experience these goals and their pursuit. Look, when I give talks I write this list on the board and then go through it. Here's what I say." I pointed to the list again and took a deep breath.

"You get good grades so you can go to a good college so you can get a good job so you can afford to borrow the money to buy a car so you can get married so you can afford to borrow the money to buy a house so you can have kids." I exhaled. They sat silently, stunned at how distasteful my summary of American life could be. I usually experienced this stunned silence when I gave talks. It hit home.

"Here's the thing. In all my interviews, these successful people wanted all of these things. They just used how they felt to make decisions about what schools, cars, spouses, homes, etc., they pursued. If you do not pay attention to how you feel, then you don't know how to make these decisions for yourself. They collected data about their own lives, about how they felt, then they put that information to work for them. They understood that how they felt pursuing the goals was as important as how they felt when they had achieved the goals. One fed the other. They found that small, but consistent buzz of energy was sustainable as long as they paid attention to it and nurtured it. And they reached these goals that we all have. They simply did not mistake the achievement of these goals as the only source of fulfillment or happiness. Success was not simply defined by these goals."

I drew two narrow lines down the middle of these goals.

Success

		Have kids
	Borrow the money to buy a house	
		Get married
	Borrow the money to buy a car	
		Get a good job
	Go to a good college	
	Get good grades in school	

"Most of us are told not only that we should achieve these goals or that they will define our success or happiness. We are subsequently told HOW to achieve them. This is really where the problem comes in. What schools are good enough? What cars are cool? What jobs sound good? How much money do we need? Other people define these for us and we accept it even if we are killing ourselves trying to achieve in this way.

"And that's bad why?" asked Mark.

"Bad is probably too strong of a word. Look at the two lines I've just drawn. They create that path others want you to take. What do you see?"

"It seems very narrow," Mark replied.

"Exactly. What if it turns out there are lots of ways of achieving these same goals, ways that might fit you better? Why would you stick to this one way of doing it?"

"You're saying that these people you interviewed found a wider path to achieve these goals?" Andy asked.

"Right. They found careers and work they loved doing."

"How'd they do that?" they all asked at the same time.

"By figuring out how they wanted to feel and going after it in a responsible way," Bob smiled as he said this. He looked at me for a nod of approval. I nodded. "Most of us are never told to factor in how we feel into the equation. And yet everyone I know agrees that how we feel impacts how we perform. They also did not see achieving these goals as the source of fulfillment by themselves.

"I can sum it up with three simple points. Bob, I have not shared this with you yet." A look of betrayal shot across his face. I had hurt his feelings. He'd get over it soon enough.

"First and foremost, acknowledge that how you feel matters, that it impacts how you perform and accept responsibility for feeling the way you want to feel.

"Second, collect data. That is what the process is about—collecting data about how you want to feel, how to create that feel, and how to protect it.

"Third, put that feel to work. One of the guys I interviewed told me that he had found his passion and put it to work. He did so as an athlete and as a realtor in Maui and is successful in both worlds. I liked that. You don't have to use the word passion. We all have our own way of articulating it.

"If you do those three things, you can widen the path you take to these goals or whatever goals you decide you want to pursue."

"So why doesn't everybody live that way?" asked Lisa.

"I think that if they have tried, they have been told, by people who don't know any better, that it is a selfish way to live. They are told all their lives to be responsible. They are trained to seek security and safety. They do what others tell them. In doing that, they stop being themselves and let others define their worlds. Then they wonder why they are unhappy or feel empty. It goes back to society. This country was built from scratch. It required people to focus on gaining freedom from the elements and from tyrants.

"We've come a long way since then. We're free from a lot of things, but we don't yet know how to exercise our freedom. Our educational systems still focus on minimal requirements, so people can have a job and take care of themselves. We get trained in some skill so we can make a living. The rest of our life revolves about maintaining that.

We're never really educated about how to move beyond that. The process I am describing is about exercising our freedom, enjoying it. People lose sight of all the experiences they had as kids that felt great. They lose their sense of wonder about things. Curiosity is diminished. I just help put wonder and curiosity back into their lives."

"Man, you're making me think I've wasted the last twenty years of my life," said Mark.

"No, that's not right. You have a house, a family, some money in the bank, a well-paying job. Those are all sources of freedom for you. The question is, how do you experience those things? Do they free you more often than they burden you? If not, why not? I would argue that you've lost the sense of freedom, because once you had those things you didn't know how to use them to feel more free and connected. Lisa, you're married right?"

"Yeah, 10 years."

"What did it feel like when you first fell in love?"

"It was awesome. I wanted to call him all the time, spend every minute with him."

"Then what happened?"

"Reality struck. The feelings changed, especially once we got married. Sometimes I wish I were single. But I also don't want to be alone."

"So being in love initially is like being in the zone. The truth is we don't know how to make someone fall in love, or even get that feeling back. I'm not sure I want science to ever figure out how to make someone fall in love. But there were certain conditions that felt great. What happened when the feelings changed?"

"We both thought something was wrong. We worried we had made the wrong decision in getting married."

"That's what happens to a lot of people. They love that new feeling, that attraction to an exalted, has-no-flaws other person. But as it fades, you start seeing the person for who he or she really is. The sad part is that you start noticing all the once invisible things that are wrong. How do you think that affects the relationship?"

Andy chimed "You spend less time together. You start paying attention to all the other things you might have neglected in your life. Some distance develops."

"And why don't people just get out then?"

"Because they don't want to be alone or feel as though they failed," Bob said, speaking for the first time in a while. Sounded like we needed to talk about his marriage soon.

"Exactly. So the relationship settles into avoiding failure and not wanting to be alone. All that happened, because the initial feeling of infatuation has diminished. We focus on what's wrong, and try to avoid it. The people I talked to don't live that way. What they do is to remind themselves of what is right for them, what makes it possible to feel in love again, even if for just for short periods. They do what they can to protect what's right.

"My own opinion is that a lasting marriage is about intimate friendship. Friendship can last forever. Keeping it intimate allows the infatuation to happen when it can. I mean emotional and physical intimacy. Being the real you. I learned all this too late to save my own marriage."

I took a risk in saying I was divorced. People too often assume that because I understand these concepts, that I can always apply them, that I don't make mistakes. I felt a little embarrassed and waited for them to comment. They were thinking about their own lives, though, and my embarrassment passed.

Vulnerability

"Alright. I know what you're talking about when it comes to relationships, but how do you apply that notion to the rest of life?" Lisa wondered.

"It's not applying it to your life. It is life. Think about all the things you've tried in life. Each time, there is an initial experience that maybe something is pretty good. Some of these experiences seem pretty common for people: piano or guitar lessons, sports, wanting to be a lawyer or doctor or fire chief. When we're growing up we have lots of ideas. We all want to be the rock star or star athlete or President of the United States. We want those things because we see them on television or we read about them. They're famous, and they seem to have pretty good lives. That captures our attention. Then we set out trying to be those things. By the third or fourth guitar lesson, we've given up, because the experience doesn't match our idea. It doesn't feel right. It feels like work.

"In high school, we work to get into a good college. In college, we work to get a degree so we can get a good job. But these experiences are limiting, and the number and quality of the ideas we have about what we want to do for a living are limited too. We go look for the jobs we are trained for, and we make decisions based on the salaries we can command. But too many people choose among a group of not so well formed ideas.

"What is really demanding their attention at that decision point is the reality of having to be on their own. At first it feels freeing, exciting. The first apartment, the first new car, freedom. The freedom, however, is inadequate because it is merely an exchange of one responsibility for another. Pretty soon, too many external things are demanding our attention. Responsibilities mounts as we move from dependence on our parents to dependence on our jobs. It is really a lateral move. I would argue that this all happens because we don't educate people, we train them."

"What's the difference?" asked Bob.

"I once read of a good way to distinguish between education and training. Training prepares you to avoid surprise; education prepares you to deal with surprise. When I asked the surgeons I worked with what the difference was between the good surgeons and the great ones, they gave me similar answer. Great surgeons go into every case knowing they don't know everything, but they are prepared to deal with the unknown. Bob that is why I am hoping that what you learn is not what someone like Jeff knows, but how they know it. It is a dynamic process."

"So what this boils down to is that we have a lot of ideas that we test out as kids, but don't really stick with them. Why do we do that?" asked Mark.

"I think we have ideas that may have a pretty attractive end result, but doing the work to get us there doesn't resonate with us. We don't gain energy from them, and we turn away. Then as we get older, the demands of taking care of ourselves, of being responsible, diminish our curiosity and our free time so we stop looking. Actually we become less vulnerable to new ideas."

"What do you mean by vulnerable?" asked Andy.

"Think about it. You all go to movies, right? You go in, get the popcorn, soda. You kick back in your chair, and you wait for the movie to start. In essence, you are making yourself vulnerable to the movie, open to its message. If you know it is about something you like, you're even more vulnerable. You let the movie come to you. If it's well done, it engages you.

"The best movies engage you, because the experiences of the characters are either similar to yours, or experiences you wish you could have. The movie ends, and you walk away pumped or sad or calm, depending on what the director was after. The theater is a place you can go and be safe to open up. The risk of opening up to a movie is small. So you go in and allow yourself to be vulnerable. The people who make movies and design theaters know that. That is why they have put the drink holders and reclining seats, to help you to be vulnerable to the movie. The less comfortable you are, the more likely you will be distracted and shut down."

"I see." Bob was a step ahead of me. "So when you go to a movie you prepare to be vulnerable, to experience and enjoy the movie."

"Right. Let's take the scenario a little further. You hear from all your friends that there is this great movie in town. You're excited to go see it. Or maybe you've read the book, and can't wait to see the movie. You're excited going in. You watch the movie and about half way through it, you realize you're bored or maybe even angry. Same movie everyone else saw, but you can't enjoy it. It is because you are not vulnerable to it, because you have your own idea of what it should be. Your expectations are too strong. You blame the movie, curse the director, and go back and blast your friends. The truth is that it is your fault. You didn't let the movie come to you. You didn't experience the movie as the director intended it. In a sense, you have dangerous information about the movie going in."

"I think I see how this relates to the process," said Bob. "The process begins with ideas. Some of those ideas capture our attention because we're open to them and they engage us. That feels great, that sense of engagement. So we pursue these ideas, believing that this sense of fulfillment or engagement will just happen naturally, if we are expressing that idea." Bob was on a roll.

"Very good. But what usually happens is that the level at which some idea is performed or expressed in front of you might set you up for disappointment. If you heard Eric Clapton play the guitar or saw Michael Jordan play hoops, or watched someone at work makes the computer sing, it is exciting, captivating. You think 'Wow, I'd love to do that.' So you go buy the guitar or sign up to play hoops in a league. But right away, you realize that you have a lot to learn. It doesn't feel so engaging when your guitar doesn't sound like Clapton's, or you can't make the lay-up.

"In those realms, the cost of quitting is acceptable. You sell the guitar back to the store, or you put the new Nike Jordan's on the shelf. You realize that you ain't like Mike. But here's the dangerous part. The guy who makes the computer sing at work sucks you in. When you act on an idea that affects your livelihood, the cost of quitting is much higher. So you learn, you practice, and you acquire some skills. But the sense of engagement has disappeared. You can't just quit because you need to eat. So you spend the rest of your life in front of a terminal."

They were all looking down and shuffling their feet. Lisa was swirling the beer around her glass.

"That's depressing because it sounds so familiar. What the hell do you do about that," whispered Andy.

"Actually it's pretty simple and doable, but it takes guts. You start just as Bob has. You start looking for the simple places where you can engage. My experience with people is that these moments do exist. The problem is that the people are not vulnerable to them anymore. They are caught up in holding onto the power they have, their ability to make money, to perform at their job, things like that. Going back to the movie analogy, it means finding and creating those moments in your life where you can be vulnerable."

"That sounds really weak."

"Unless you remember what I said about the surgeons. It is preparing to deal with surprise not avoiding it. That takes courage."

A grin broke out across Bob's face. "That's the preparation stage of the process."

"Being vulnerable is important at every stage of the model," I corrected Bob. "In order to know what your dream is, how you want life to feel, you have to be open to it. You have to pay attention to the places engagement happens. Who does it happen around? How does it happen? What things can you control? The preparation stage is then trying things on, seeing if there is a good fit for you."

"I hate to say this, but I have to run. I have to finish some stuff up at the office," said Mark. He chugged the remains of his beer and offered his hand to me. "Thanks. I still have questions for you, though. Same time next week?"

Lisa agreed. "Yeah, can we do this again?"

Andy just nodded. I agreed to meet with them again soon. Bob was beaming as we walked out to the cars.

"That was fun!" Bob gushed. "I must admit I was having my doubts, because I couldn't answer all of their questions."

"No problem. Look, Bob, I've been doing this a while, and it took me a long time to be able to understand it and articulate it. Keep in mind, though that I am not always going to be there to answer the questions or to help you ask the right questions. That is up to you. I'll be out of town the next couple of weeks. I want you to go meet with this guy." I handed him a piece of paper with a name and a number on it.

"John Molo. Your drummer friend. He'll talk with me?"

"Sure. You can learn a lot of from him. He has thought a great deal about how he wants to live his life. He works as hard as anyone I've ever met to hold onto his own ideas and to his dreams about what music means to him. He wants to create and express his own ideas musically. He does it in a very unforgiving arena. The music business is brutal. He balances his ideas with the demands of the public and the demands of the music business. He makes himself vulnerable to his own ideas and at the same time he is vulnerable to the powers that be. He is very good at achieving that balance. He prepares as well anyone I've ever met. He can do that because he is very clear about what music gives him. As a drummer, he really has to make himself vulnerable to the needs of the other musicians he plays with."

"He sounds great. I'll go see him. Where are you going?"

"I have to give a talk in Hawaii, but most of the time while I'm there I'll be playing: rollerblading, body surfing, biking."

"Sounds rough."

"Believe me, Bob. I've done a lot of work and been through a lot to get to the point that someone will pay me to talk. Preparation. What will you work for?"

"Got it." He walked away deep in thought. The thought of calling Molo intimidated him. I knew he'd be fine. Molo is a good guy.

Maui

Ah! Maui. I had left Charlottesville a day early because a huge snowstorm was due the day I was scheduled to leave. I had an extra day to enjoy before the conference was to start. I had negotiated a Jeep Wrangler for the week I was there, as part of my fee. Maui was completely different than Waikiki where I had been with the basketball team ten years earlier. Waikiki was more like New York City with sun. I'm not complaining. We had a blast each year we went there, but Maui was more my style. As I drove along the beach, I saw hordes of surfers sitting on their boards waiting, hoping, for that next big set to come in. I promised myself that someday I would learn how to surf.

I pulled up to the hotel, checked in, and went to the room. I opened the blinds to an incredible view of the surf crashing onto the volcanic shore. Out the front window, other tourists whose white skin reflected the sun, much as mine, surrounded the pool. I unpacked, which for me simply means opening my suitcase. I grabbed my running shoes and rollerblades. I decided running was a wiser choice given the hills I had seen driving into the hotel. Just outside the hotel was a running path that snaked along the shoreline. I pulled on my shoes and shorts and headed towards the path.

Whenever I experience something remarkable, my first instinct is to want to share it with someone. My divorce had finalized several years earlier, then went through another difficult breakup, and now dated casually. I wasn't ready for a committed relationship, though. I needed to know myself better, and enjoyed being alone on special trips like this. I was good at being alone at home, but the excitement of a new place left me longing.

I ran along the winding path. Huge waves crashed in front of the hotel. Red flags dotted the coast indicating the surf was too dangerous for swimming. I noticed people snorkeling in a small, protected cove. I added that to my list of things to do while I was there. There were couples walking on the beach holding hands. That made me feel good about someday sharing the good things in my life with someone. I have some incredible friendships in my life, and they are always there when I need them. They have really helped me through the tough times, but the feeling of sharing the best things in my life is something I am saving for one person, whoever that might be. Until that happens, though, my friends and my self-resilience are more than enough to help me live the life I want.

Upset Of The Century

As I ran, it was hard to avoid thinking back to my college years. Hawaii was the big event of the year. We were away from our families and friends on Christmas morning. But it never felt like Christmas being in Hawaii, so we didn't feel we were missing something.

I laughed as I remembered my senior year. We played Georgetown with Patrick Ewing the night before leaving for Tokyo. Ralph Sampson, our perennial player of the year and seven-foot-four center had come down with a bad case of the flu. Sports Illustrated called it the Game of the Century. I played one second in front of my hometown crowd. *One second.* We won and Ralph outplayed Ewing despite his illness. Othell Wilson and Ricky Stokes, the guards, played extremely well.

On the plane to Japan, Ralph was attached to an IV to keep his fluids up. We had just played in Tokyo against Houston and Utah and beaten them both. When we got to Japan, he couldn't play no matter how much the president of Suntory Beer, the game's sponsor, begged him to. No one thought we had a chance of beating Houston without Ralph, who had Clyde Drexler and Akeem Olajuwon, but we beat them easily.

We left Tokyo to fly to Hawaii on a Monday night, passed the International Date Line, and arrived in Waikiki on Monday morning. Our body clocks were all out of whack. Tuesday night we went bar hopping and ran into the number-one ranked women's team in the country. Cheryl Miller, the best player in the country, starred for them. The focus of most of the guys on the team, however, was on Pam and Paula McGee, twins who were about six-foot tall. They were especially good looking. At the bar, several of the guys on the team danced and left with some of the USC players. I left alone. I had met a cheerleader in Tokyo from the University of Utah, and I couldn't get her out of my mind.

The next night in Waikiki, we played an NAIA school, Chaminade. We were the number-one ranked team, the best team in the country. Chaminade was so small, they weren't even in the NCAA. They played out of their minds and beat us by one point. We were shocked. The truth is, I had mostly stopped caring about things like this, because I never played and felt that what I did had little bearing on the team's success. Even so, it was a shocker.

Coach Holland told us to have fun the rest of the trip, and we would deal with the loss later. That's exactly what I did. The next morning I woke up and tried to call home. In a faint voice ghosting over from another line I heard someone say, "It was the upset of the century." I just laughed while my call was still going through. From the Game of the Century to the Upset of the Century within one week's time. Fifteen years later people still ask me if I was on the team that lost to Chaminade.

My mind drifted back to the present as I ran. I thought about how much I had changed, how I could see those college years so differently now than when they were actually happening. The time I had worked through the process over the past years had allowed me to see what basketball had meant to me, what mistakes I had made, and given me the hope to avoid them in the future.

What do I know now that I didn't know then? Basketball in high school was engaging. I loved putting in the hours, discovering and enjoying my talent. My coach was a hard nose who had no problem yelling and screaming at me. Though I can't say I loved it, I never took it personally. He challenged me honestly and directly. Then he gave me the opportunity to prove myself. Basketball was the perfect place for me to balance my desire and my fear. It was on the basketball court that the standing civil war became a competition, two forces pushing against each other creating energy, excitement, and the right amount of doubt to compel me to improve.

Fortunately, I was a good enough athlete to rise to his challenges, even if it took time. My junior year, he deliberately put me on the third team the first day of practice. I was the best player coming back from the previous year, yet I was third string. I was pissed every day I went to practice. I never considered accepting it or backing off. He called me names and challenged me in front of the other players, but I was able to stay engaged in the practices.

Looking back, I can see that it was because I loved playing so much. I had already learned how to really push myself running in the off-season and doing drills into the late hours of the night. I pushed myself because I would rather being doing those things than anything else. I also never felt my coach was trying to take something away from me. Maybe I just felt he couldn't take it away.

Make Tomorrow Better Than Today

Years later, I interviewed National Defensive Player of the Year, Tommy Ammaker. He was then an assistant coach at Duke, and he is now the head coach of Seton Hall's basketball team. We had a discussion about players who don't play much. I'll never forget what he told me. He said that at Duke, they never talked about playing time. He said his responsibility to the players was to help them get better as players everyday. Period. There is only so much playing time available and talking about it really doesn't accomplish much. Talking about it certainly didn't make anyone better. The only way to get playing time was to earn playing time. To do that, the only thing in the player's control was to get better.

When my high school coach put me on the third string, I trusted him enough to believe that if I kept getting better, he would have a hard time keeping me on the bench. I dealt with it simply by engaging more deeply in the playing. Practice was a serious competition for me, everyday the equivalent of a real game. I pushed others hard in practice. I was in the best shape of my life, and I was getting a lot better. The night of the first game I walked into the locker room and saw my name at the top of the board. I ended up being the only player who started every game that year, and I was named player of the year.

Drifting back out of my reminiscing, my legs were tiring, and I was really far from the hotel. A luau was starting near the beach. I saw that the group was obviously a sales organization's quota club, and I chuckled at them in their Hawaiian shirts ogling the dancers. I took off my shirt and shoes and sprinted into the waves. I caught a couple of waves, once actually body surfing into the curl and riding the wave parallel to the beach. That was breathtaking. Easy Speed. Rouse had taught me a little about playing in the water. I walked out and sat in the sand where the water line could hit my feet.

College had not been as easy for me. Basketball tapped into all the adoption issues for me. In high school, my coach had been like a father for me. Not that I needed one, but I certainly still sought fatherly approval from him. When I didn't get it, I knew how to go about it. He was always very clear about what he expected from me. No matter how harshly he may have delivered the message, I understood it, because I wanted to do things right for him and for myself.

My college coach was much more reserved and somewhat distant. At the time I played for him, I felt ignored. That was, and still is, the worst thing someone can do to me. When it involves something as important to me as basketball was, and relationships still are, being ignored causes that pain in my stomach to churn full tilt. I have always felt able to defend myself when attacked, but feeling that I don't count leaves me defenseless and weak.

Four years of never knowing where I stood in his eyes, or what I had to do, totally drained me. I stopped focusing on being better, on engaging in my dream, even of the joy of playing. My focus went straight to minutes of playing time, and I bought into all the dull and predictable comments that people made around me. They just kept asking why wasn't I playing. I fixated on that and blamed the coach. Worst of all, the feelings of being ignored seemed to confirm what being adopted had taught me. I wasn't important. I didn't count. I would never be good enough and there was nothing I could do.

My most notable moments as a college player never seemed to happen on the court. I was a sideshow act. Somehow I was mentioned in Sports Illustrated three times for off-court rather than on-court actions: for having pet snakes that would start in my locker and show up in someone else's, for doing funny things in practice, and for playing horse before the game with fans. I am still remembered in the equipment room for the fact that as a senior my name was misspelled "Newbury" on my jersey for the opening game of the season against the Russian Olympic team. Before the game I pointed this out to my coach, and he said no one would notice but my parents. As I went into the game, the announcer said, "Now entering the game, number 32, Doug Newbury." My parents and 10,000 other people noticed. For the rest of the year friends sent mail and made checks out to Doug Newbury.

My most memorable moment in University Hall happened in our last home game as seniors. Ralph, Craig Robinson, and I had been called back on the court for a post game ceremony. The P.A. Announcer was reading Ralph's list of accomplishments as he received an award from the Governor. "Three time All-American, Three time National Player of the Year, Leading rebounder in Virginia history..." I couldn't resist. I raised my arms above my head, pretending they were describing me. The crowd fell apart. It was as close as I came to a moment of glory.

Sometimes in life, a single act can neatly characterize a longer experience. That happened when I got married. For my wedding, Coach and his wife gave Annie and me pewter Jefferson cups with the date of our wedding engraved just below our names. When I read the inscription, I fell on the floor laughing. Annie asked me what was wrong? I handed her the cup and she, too, burst out laughing. Instead of "Doug and Annie," the cup read "Dud and Annie." They wanted us to exchange them, but that would have been dishonest. As far as my basketball career went, the engraver could not have said it better.

I glanced up. The sun had started to set. It was magnificent. I wondered what it would be like to live here, to see this spectacular sight everyday. Then I remembered the sunsets in Free Union and realized what I had was just as good, simply different. I started back for the hotel, a little worked up about my college memories. Years earlier, I would have had nightmares about it. The recurring nightmare was being locked out of the arena while the team was playing North Carolina. I would sprint around trying every door. Finally, the coach would open one and just laugh, then shut it in my face.

Now, though, I understand the pain of all of these things, particularly the pain the adoption caused. I can express it to myself and differentiate between the present and the past. I can learn from the past instead of reliving it. I can live in the present even if my past tries to haunt me. That knowledge allows me to prepare for what's next without giving into the baggage of the past. I'm not saying I am perfect at this, but I miss fewer opportunities in my life now.

I also know more about what I want and what I will work for in my life. I understand the settings in which I can be myself. I know what situations will challenge me, or threaten what's right about me, and I can prepare better to deal with them by improving, not by withdrawing.

The mistake I made in choosing a college is right at the heart of the dream-goal distinction. I chose college for external reasons: television, prestige, championships, in short for basketball, not for an education, and for the wrong basketball reasons at that. I knew that playing at Virginia was not a guarantee. I was not a "can't miss" prospect. In fact, I was not one of Virginia's first choices. I based my decision on factors I had no control over. Sure, I could get better, but being on television and playing in the ACC had never been important to me until others kept talking about it. I guess I was afraid of not getting to play at that level. Even my high school coach thought I should go there.

My dream was to play, to engage in each shot, each dribble, each game. I had lost sight that of that. At some level, I was reminded of that loss everyday in practice, every time I felt like I didn't matter, whenever someone important ignored me. Sure some people would tell me how lucky I was, just getting to be a member of the team. But after every game, the athletic director would walk around the locker room and shake hands with guys who played, walking past my locker without saying a word. The truth is I didn't matter.

I could feel hurt by the athletic director, the coach, the media, or the fans. The bottom line was that I had hurt myself. What had been important to me didn't matter to me enough to protect it, to hold onto it, to work for it. How can I possibly look back and blame those people for doing the same thing I did to myself?

I continued my beach path run, and my legs reached out in a comfortable cadence, my feet bouncing off the pavement gently, my momentum forward minimizing the impact on my knees. A scene from a nineties' television show, *I'll Fly Away*, plays in my mind. The show was about Lily Harper, a black housekeeper who worked for a white family in the south in the early sixties. Lily returned home late one night to discover that her elderly father was missing. She could not find him anywhere. Eventually, she finds him in an old baseball field that is dimly lit by a single bulb. She parks the car and starts walking towards her father.

Down on the field, he stood at home plate wielding an old 2x4 board as though it were his favorite Louisville Slugger. He concentrates on the mound, hoping the imaginary pitcher will put a fastball right down the middle. He swings the bat, makes a cracking sound with his mouth, and takes off around the bases. As he crosses first base he realizes that the ball has carried past the run-down fence for a home run. He jumps high in the air, raising his arms above his head, palms open to receive the praise of the crowd. His pace slows to a home-run trot. He takes his time to enjoy the moment and to let the pitcher know who won that round.

As he approaches home plate, he realizes that his angry and bewildered daughter is waiting to scold him. He is brought crashing back to the reality, like a small child who knows he has done something wrong. He never does touch home plate.

"Daddy, What is wrong with you? Have you lost your mind?" Asks Lily.

Her father pauses. Suddenly, his look changes from someone being scolded to someone with something important to say. A touch of anger flashes across his eyes only to be replaced by the caring look of a wise father.

"Daughter, let me tell you something. When I was a ball player back in the old Negro Leagues, I had a certain something that I'm missing now. I didn't really understand until tonight. When I played ball, everything I did mattered. If I swung at the ball or if I didn't swing at the ball, it mattered. If I caught the ball in the outfield or if it got by, it mattered. I miss that feeling. I like it when what I do matters, when I matter."

This TV show is another coin in my mind's jar of loose change. Rather than trying to understand the characteristics of the people who choose to perform, I wanted to know what compelled people to action and turned reactors into performers. Performers deliberately put themselves in situations in which everything matters. Curt Tribble has an explicit credo of "Everything Matters." Performers enjoy that pressure. They thrive on it. I believed that about myself.

I got back to the hotel under the moonlight. The crashing sound told me the waves were getting bigger. I felt myself letting go of the past reminders of basketball in Hawaii. The process of focusing on my own role in my earlier emotional demise, gave me part of the means to deal with it. I felt a sense of control, of knowing what I needed to do.

My life as a speaker and as someone who works with others reminds me so much of the early days when I played basketball for the right reasons. My life now is like that game of basketball. I can't control the outcome. I work to make the audience understand, but sometimes they don't. I work to help the person come to grips with their inner capacity, but sometimes they can't. What I can do is to keep improving, keep listening to and learning from others, and then keep testing myself. I had to talk in two days. I looked forward to it the same way I went into my high school games: excited, uncertain of what would happen, but with the belief that I could make a difference, because I was well prepared. I had done the work and I knew if it didn't come out exactly right, I could learn from it without beating myself up and withdrawing.

Chapter 6

A Dream Deferred

Engaging Vacations

"Nice tan," Bob teased.

"Makes me feel healthy."

"Yeah, I guess two weeks in Hawaii will do that." He walked in and sat down in my office.

"Have you ever been there?" I asked him.

"Yeah, but it was a nightmare. That long plane ride. Taking vacations is difficult for me."

"Why?"

"Well, I'm always stressed getting ready for them. When I get where I'm going, I spend the first few days worrying about what's going on in the office. I'm always checking my messages. By the third day, I relax a little bit, but I feel as though I have to make sure everyone else is having a good time. By the end of the trip, I begin to worry about what is waiting for me at the office. We always get back from vacations late the Sunday before I have to start work again. I come into the office, I'm not looking forward to it, and I'm tired. The trip to Hawaii is even harder because of the time differences. Then I spend two weeks catching up."

"So why do you take vacations?" I wondered.

"Well, I avoid them if I can. It's just easier to keep working. But my family needs them, and I do spend some time with them."

"What would you like the vacations to feel like?"

"Relaxed. I always thought of vacations as a way of escaping, of getting away, but it doesn't seem to feel that way."

"Given what we've talked about, what would be a more useful way to think about them?"

"Good question!" He sat and thought for a while.

"Suppose I changed your word escape to disengage?" I asked.

"What do you mean?"

"Well, do you really want to disengage from your life?"

"I hadn't thought of that. No, I guess not."

"So how do you take a vacation to engage in your life, not escape it?"

"I would start by knowing how I want it to feel. My vacations are built on the notion of freedom from. You're saying I should seek the freedoms to and of the vacation."

"I'm not saying anything. I'm asking you how you want your vacations to feel. If you weren't married or working and you went to Hawaii for a week, what would you do?"

"I'd play more. I'd learn to windsurf. I'd play golf, run on the beach, bike."

"Why would you do those things?"

"Because they would engage me." He laughed.

"And you blame your wife, your kids, your job for the way your vacations feel?"

"I guess I do. Remember when I first came to you. I said I wanted to be able to do something for myself. I guess that is what vacations should be."

"So why do you have a wife, and kids, and a job?"

"Don't get me wrong. I love my family. I even like my job. Sometimes they just keep me from living the way I want to live."

"A month ago you couldn't even tell me how you wanted to live. Do you know now?"

"I'm getting there. I want to engage in my life. I want to feel a sense of freedom. I like being engaged in solving problems and in helping other people. I like being creative. I've also discovered that when I'm engaged in my life, there is a flow to it, a certain rhythm."

"And when does that happen?"

"Mostly when I'm doing something with others, or when I'm playing like when we did the motorcycles. At work, it's when I can dive into a project or work on solving a problem. It happens best when I can think something through and then pass on the more technical work to the people who like doing that sort of thing. Most of the time on our projects involves other people. Molo got me thinking about that."

"How was Johnnie Mo?"

Bob laughed. "I had a great time with him. He made me feel so important around him. If it weren't for the gold records hanging on his wall, I would never have known he was as distinguished a musician as he is."

"I love Johnnie Mo. He has this energy about him."

"That's exactly right," Bob agreed. "A genuineness. Authentic. I liked talking to him, because as a drummer he isn't the star of the group, but he has an important effect on the final outcome and the experience of the other players."

"What did you learn from him?"

"Nothing new, but he made some ideas clearer for me. The first was something that I know you've mentioned before. I have had trouble getting over the notion that working on myself was selfish, but Molo talked about how his role is to make others better. He said that he wants to be the kind of guy that people would say is great to work with. Not in a way that he is self-deprecating. How'd he say it? Something like he didn't need to have the fastest hands or loudest cymbals, but that he can interact with the other players in a civil manner and draw the best out of them, while he maintained his own integrity and dignity. I'd love it if someone described me like that."

"Does that sound selfish?"

"Not at all. He also talked about his theory of trying less. He talked about how we're taught to try hard. He made a distinction between working hard and trying hard. He said when you're trying hard, you're really not trying. If you know you're trying to force something to happen, you're not trusting what you know and letting it happen. When he plays really well, it's because he has done the hard work in the preparation and then he just takes advantage of it. He lets it happen.

"He was really into the preparation, doing the mental, physical, and emotional work. I remembered something you and I talked about when you asked me if I knew what my boss wanted from me. It never occurred to me that I should really know anything other than what he *told* me he wanted. John told me though about how when Hornsby talked about the music he liked, John would go listen to it and learn how to play it. Bruce never asked him to do it. Knowing that music made it easier for Bruce and John to work together. John had some idea of the things Bruce liked."

"I remember him telling me that, too," I said. "It's a good point. In the music world, it would be hard for Bruce to articulate what it was about a certain style or piece of music that grabbed him. John listened to the music and learned to play it so they could experience it together. My guess is that your boss couldn't articulate certain things to you either. By paying attention and taking responsibility, you might figure out something he wants but can't articulate, that only shows up in the way he behaves."

"Right," Bob agreed. "Molo made some good points about supporting the leader of any group. The time he spent with Bruce, he felt responsible for getting things off to a good start. He said that a person should try hard to make the leader believe that the person can contribute, can help fulfill the group's dreams. The leader needs to know that you're behind him. I certainly have not done a very good job of that at work. I think my relationship with my boss is based too much on fear.

"I asked John what I should do about that. Basically he said to learn as much as possible about the big picture that the boss sees and then focus on the smaller pieces that I can help with. Molo was very clear, though, about doing it in a way that is consistent with my own values and beliefs. He said that he couldn't go out on stage and not be true to his own style. He used the words 'honoring the song.' I don't think I honor my work enough. I just go through the motions."

"Good observation."

"The other thing he mentioned was expanding your circle of influences. Seek out talented, effective people. That sounds to me like what you've done."

"It is. At one point in my graduate program, I felt bored. Sport psychology is not exactly brain surgery. My dad told me that I needed to seek out people in other fields, to engage in an intellectual conversation about performance, to test my thinking against first-rate minds. I've been lucky that I have been able to collaborate with such people in the hospital and in the business school.

"Again, though, I was prepared when the opportunities presented themselves. If I hadn't known how to interact, or if I tried to sell myself as an expert, they would have laughed me out of the place. I deliberately listened to people for a long time. I looked for a fit, instead of just forcing my way in. I developed relationships, had conversations. I learned from them, and in return they were willing to listen to what I had to say."

"I think I can apply those ideas to my relationships with customers and my colleagues in other departments," said Bob. "Then when problems or opportunities come up, the relationships are already in place."

"You might broaden out and make some new friends as well. That is certainly what happened to me."

"One idea John shared made me question my own behavior. He told me a story about auditioning a new bass player for a band he played in. He said the guy came out and just wasn't making it. John nicely told him that he didn't get the gig. Immediately, the guy started making excuses. John sat and listened to him and wanted to say, 'You just weren't good enough,' but he didn't. Molo asked me how I would deal with a situation like that. Unfortunately, I realized that I would have done the same thing that musician did. I would have taken it personally and become defensive. So John pointed out that seeing yourself as a whole person, and not labeling yourself as a drummer or an athlete or computer guy, is an important way to deal with those situations. Maybe the gig wasn't right. Maybe he needed to practice, to learn more."

"I run into that a lot in the work I do," I added. "One way to think about it is to improve yourself, to build on what's right. Too many people merely focus on what's wrong and try to fix it. That's a recipe for disaster, because you slowly lose confidence and forget all the other things you have to offer the world."

"I do that all the time," Bob said. "I just beat myself up over and over and over. Then I get mad at my boss or my wife for making me feel bad. John made me realize that being told I messed up and getting specific information is really a gift. If people just let me continue doing mediocre work, they aren't doing me a favor. It's tough. John talked about high school, and how bad a student he felt he was. He knew that his band teacher really believed in him. He said that was a big part of his drive and success."

I replied, "That's George Horan alright. Actually he had a role in reuniting me with Molo. I saw a video on MTV of Hornsby's 'The Way It Is' and I thought it was great. They played at the Warner Theater so I went to check them out. I looked up on stage and saw George Horan. I wondered how this old guy from my high school had hooked up with Hornsby. Later in the show, Bruce introduced the band. He got to the drummer and said, 'From McLean, Virginia, John Molo.' I couldn't believe it. John and I had lost track of each other when I went to college. So I wrote to him and we've been good friends ever since."

"Yes," Bob replied, "John told me he had run into George a few weeks before the gig. He reminded George that he had been a lousy student. George told him he was the best student he ever had. Molo struggled not to cry when he was telling me that. Molo told me that Horan would come into class every once in a while and say he had played at a local bar, and say he had played with some rising stars. He specifically mentioned the day Horan came in and told them to go buy all the James Brown records they could because he had played with James Brown the night before at the Howard Theater."

"Someone once asked Horan why he was a teacher," I recalled. "He said 'I'm not a teacher. I'm a musician who teaches.' Molo loved that. I would say that about most of the people I interviewed. They love to teach what they know best and have a passion about. It is not so much teaching the information as sharing their passion."

"Yes, I want to do that with my family. Molo got me thinking about who I influence, and the opportunities I have to pass on things to people around me. I need to start with my family. I need to figure out what I want in life. Then I need to ask my wife what she wants in life. What do you think?"

I leaned forward and thought for a moment, trying to decide whether or not to answer this for Bob. Was he seeking information or my approval? I believed Bob was past looking for my approval, that he wanted to know what I thought. I trusted that he would consider what I had to say, and not simply do what I said.

The Real Competition

"Bob, You can't make good decisions unless you have good information. If you have been living your life to avoid certain things, merely to fulfill responsibilities, how do you think the people around you are living? Bruce Hornsby gave me his philosophy about his life and his career. It seems relevant to this discussion. He said that 60% of his life is about being the baddest mother in music, and the remaining 40% is trying to get along with others while doing that. He said it can be trying at times, but that it is really worth it.

"In that field, he often plays with different musicians. He spends time observing and talking with the musicians about what they are after musically. In live performances, he seems to give each of the band members something they can hold onto for themselves. He has a vision musically of what he's after, but he gives the other band members the room and freedom to express their own ideas. He said that ultimate freedom for him is when he goes on this musical adventure with the other band members.

"He spends a lot of time honing his skills, so that his skill level rarely prevents him from trying new things or expressing new ideas. He called it 'shedding,' putting in the time (after an old shed behind his home, where he practiced piano, hours on end, months on end). He surrounds himself with musicians and engineers who are willing to put in the work and can share his musical adventure. He even built his own studio at his new home. If he has an idea in the middle of the night, he can run down and get it on tape and not lose the idea. It is preparation. What do you think he is preparing to do?"

"I always thought professional musicians enjoyed the life of a musician. The fame, the recognition, the money," Bob said tentatively.

"Bruce seems to have more internal drive," I responded. "He wants to be great, but what he means by that is not what I expected. It goes back to defining performance as the creation and expression of his idea, his music. He seems very competitive, but not in the sense that he wanted to win something with his music. His competition is more internal. He is challenging his skills as a musician, as a songwriter, and as a producer to live up to the vision inside him. The challenge lies somewhere between creating an idea and expressing it. The sense of resonance, of engagement lies in the doing, not merely in the result.

"After seven-and-a-half years of trying to get a record contract, Bruce finally got one with RCA. They cut the record and he wasn't satisfied, so he spent hour after hour trying to make it better. He had to convince the record company to let him do more work on it, even though they were already happy with it. They finally released it, but he still didn't feel great about it. His true competition is between his skills and his vision. He started writing songs and producing them, because that helped get him more involved in expressing his vision. He said that publishing songs is where the real money is, but that didn't strike me as money conscious. Having the money was another form of preparation for him, a means to free him to pursue his dream. He just did not want money to be an obstacle for him.

"Once he got the deal, his focus changed. Getting a contract meant nothing if he didn't have the album he wanted. When he finished the album, and it was successful, his focus shifted to his career as a musician. But what drives him, it seems to me, is the need to create music that is an expression of him, of his influences, of the things he cares about. He also wants people to 'get' his music. It is not enough to have a vision of some new form of music, if no one understands it. He wants to connect to the audience and to the other musicians. The challenge is to stay true to his vision, and to make it accessible to the people around him. He wants to reach them through his music. How might all this apply to you?"

"I want to be myself," Bob replied, "the part of myself that I value. I want others to appreciate that part of me as well. I want to have the safety to improve myself, to improve the parts of me I don't value as much, but know are part of me. I went for a drive in the mountains the other night and thought about what I've learned so far. I did a benefit-cost analysis." He looked at me through the corners of his eyes and laughed. It was a nervous laugh. "The cost of acceptance by others is too high, if it means not being myself. The challenge is to hold onto myself--my ideas, my dreams-- and to develop the skills to be accessible to others, to invest in myself in a way that connects me with other people.

"I've tried to be independent, but I realize now that I am just disconnected. My wife doesn't really know who I am, and that's not her fault. I haven't been clear on what I want. I've developed the skills to be accepted, but that's not me. People might accept my skills and the things I produce, but the people I care about don't even know me. How can I feel accepted if I haven't even shown them myself?"

"Heavy stuff."

"Yeah, but it makes so much sense now. I've been running around trying to get people to accept me, and it has had too high a cost. The benefits just are not enough. The cost is almost always higher."

"So are you going to quit your job and get a divorce?"

"No, exactly the opposite. I want to find the places in my life that I can engage in the real me, in the part of me that I value the most. Until I can do that I can't blame other people for not giving me what I want. I'm going to go back home and spend time with my wife and help her help me. I'm going to offer to help her, however I can. I know it might be hard, but it seems to me to be worth it. I don't want a divorce. I love her. I can't imagine my life without her, but I know the life we have can be better.

"It makes me think about what it should mean when you get engaged to be married. In my case, what a joke. I didn't take it seriously. It's time to re-engage. I stopped by the jewelry store on the way home from the mountains, and I bought her a new engagement ring. This time I will really engage her." I could see the tears streaming down his face. He saw me wipe my eyes. "Sorry," he said.

"No need to be sorry."

"I feel like I have so much more to tell you, but I need a break." He looked up for permission

"Sounds good. Fifteen minutes."

"Sure. I'll be back." His sense of resolve showed in his gait. He moved slowly, but with purpose. He needed some time to think. So did I.

Sharing My Fears

I walked down the halls of the hospital and out to the Rotunda. I stood at the top stair and looked out over the Lawn to the far end. Cabel Hall was not part of Jefferson's original design. The addition blocked out the view of the mountain that Jefferson intended as a symbol of what was possible, of the future. I wondered what Jefferson would think of Cabel Hall. What would he think of higher education today?

Thomas Jefferson suffered great loss in his life. He lost several of his children and his wife to early death. At some point in his life, he decided to disregard his heart and live in his mind. Maybe that is why he didn't get issues such as slavery right. Compassion takes a connection to the heart. If he had abandoned his heart as so many of us do, how could he make compassionate decisions?

I can only imagine that the losses he suffered were overwhelming. He found distraction in a multitude of talents. But what was the cost?

Did he enjoy his talents, or were they merely a diversionary tactic to aim him away from a broken heart? I asked myself these questions, because I knew we were coming to a difficult stage of the process with Bob. The rubber would soon meet the pavement, or Bob would stop seeing me. I'd grown to like Bob. I appreciated his willingness to do the work. It is a rare quality. I had seen fear ruin too many lives, extract too high a cost from too many people.

I knew that delving into fear with someone made me too vulnerable at times, usurping my power, minimizing my skills. I knew I would have to share with Bob my fears and the true reason I do what I do.

When he came back, I said, "I was an illegitimate kid. Born to a flight attendant from Tennessee who had a one-year stand with a college kid from Catholic University. Born with twisted legs, I spent the first six months of my life in and out of the hospital in corrective care. I had a foster mother who reported I cried too much. The only other notes they could find from the doctors who cared for me, said what a good baby I was. The gap in descriptions didn't make much sense to me. All I know is the deep-seated fear I lived with for most of my life. The surgery and braces patched my legs, but I was left with a wounded heart.

"Being adopted is a strange thing. My adopted sister has none of the same fears or questions that I have. We were both raised by wonderful parents who showed us what love is. I was lucky, but not whole. For most of my life, I watched my unknown fear drive my behaviors. When I got divorced ten years ago, I knew I had to do something to change.

"As a kid in grade school I was bussed across Northern Virginia to participate in the first gifted class in the area. Twelve kids from all over coming together for 'special education.' I didn't feel special. I just felt different. The school we attended made things even worse. We were the geeks in a school of street kids.

"The first day of school, the biggest kid on the playground walked up to me smiled, said 'Hi,' and then kneed me in the groin. I threw up, and the other kids laughed. At one point, I came to school every morning and threw up on the floor. I was scared to death. I felt disconnected, alone, and out of place. I was in a class of bright kids who cared about school, but all I cared about was sports. Eventually, I got the street kids to accept me at recess, because I had a great arm and was the best player in most of our games. I lived for recess and lost all interest in schoolwork.

"In eighth grade, I had both knees operated on at the same time, with casts from waist to ankle. I would walk two miles everyday in the casts to a basketball court, and spend hours shooting by myself. When the casts were removed, I had a good enough shot to play with the best players. I could also see the playground at an elementary school from my bedroom window. I would stay there late into the evening, because my parents could see me and not worry. Basketball wasn't my first love, but it was something I could practice alone.

"I finally rejoined the neighborhood kids on entry to the local high school. The problem was I didn't know any of them. I was a just another scrawny kid with long hair. I went to school everyday and played hoops before school, at lunch, and after school. When team tryouts came around, I didn't even know what they meant. I went out because so many kids said I should. I made the freshman squad only because I out-hustled everyone else. By the end of freshman year, I was starting.

"Then something wonderful happened. I grew seven inches in one year. I kept playing after school everyday, and eventually my body and my skills caught up with my idea of basketball. As a senior, I was Player of the Year in my area and got scholarship offers. I started to think I was something special.

"I signed to play at the University of Virginia. During my years there our squad won more games over a four-year stretch than any other team in NCAA history, but I rarely played and took on the role of crowd pet. You know, the guy who comes in at the end of the blowout game that everyone cheers for. Every time I touched the ball, even if I was 90 feet away from the basket, the crowd would yell 'Shoot!' It was humiliating."

The Human Victory Cigar

"By my senior year, the crowd chants had become expected, part of the game. We won a lot of blowouts, so the crowd often got to see me play a bit. We were playing Duke and we were up by 20 or so points. The crowd wanted me in the game so they could cheer me on to shoot from some ridiculous distance.

"'Let's cheer for Newburg!' I could hear a preppily dressed, middle-aged woman suggest somewhere not too far behind me.

"'We don't have a big enough lead yet,' proclaimed her husband, whose bright orange blazer loudly declared his support for UVa. Eventually, Coach Holland put me in the game.

"The next day I picked up a copy of the Washington Post at 7-11. I sat in my car in the parking lot and pulled out the sports page. The headline read 'Virginia Trounces Duke.' The first line in the article read: 'You knew that victory was in hand when Coach Terry Holland sent in his human victory cigar, Doug Newburg.' I looked to see who had written the article: John Feinstein, drawing a parallel to Celtic Coach Red Auerbach's habit of lighting a victory cigar when a game was wrapped.

"As I moved from high school to college, my dreams of playing basketball took on new meanings, new images, and new feelings. The inspirational dreams of challenge, of playing to win, of public self-expression were replaced by the dreams of emotional safety, of anonymity, of solitude. The dreams in my mind became images of failure and rejection, constantly weighing me down. I was completely lost.

"In high school, basketball meant acceptance. People who wouldn't talk to me as a freshman actually asked for my autograph when I was a senior. I admit it felt cool, but it felt strange, surreal. The problem is I bought into it. I believed the hype. In college, what had been a source of identity in high school became a source of shame and embarrassment. People told me I was whining too much because I wanted to play. The same people laughed when I didn't get into the game.

"A few years out of college I ran into John Feinstein. He came running over and said, 'I need to apologize to you. When I wrote that about you I didn't understand.'

"'Understand what?' I asked John."

"'Look, I just spent a year at Indiana University working on a book. I spent a lot of time with the guys at the end of the bench. I didn't understand that they had the same dream as the guys on the court. The dream was to play.' "

"Before he told me that, I had never looked at playing that way. That was when it first hit me that the dream was not winning a championship. The dream was playing, the unadulterated joy of playing. As a guy at the end of the bench, I had just *practiced* basketball for four years. Having little or no impact on the outcome of the game was boring. Because of my experience in high school, I knew what it felt like to play when it mattered, to make a meaningful difference, to play to win. That was the dream."

Bob was riveted. He had joined me on the railing of the Rotunda.

"Wow. I guess I thought you never were scared of anything. I know that's not fair of me, but you just seem so together when we talk. I had no idea."

"Thanks. That's the danger in doing what I do. We've spent a lot of time talking about the dream and about things that might inspire you. I didn't need to share my dreams with you because you needed to find your own dream. But we're stepping to the edge of the cliff now. I felt you needed to know more about me to trust me enough to step off."

"What do you mean?" Bob asked.

"The idea is to keep your desires greater than your fears whenever possible and whenever healthy. What we've been doing is finding the desire inside of you and in your life. We're looking for your freedoms and joys. Those are what will give you the courage to work on the fear side of the equation. If we just work on the desire side, you'll eventually burn out. The fears never go away. You just avoid them. Then when you're doing something really important, they'll show up and trivialize all the work you've done. We need to find a reason for you to want to do the real work: to face your fears."

"That sounds horrible."

"Well, it's not as bad as it sounds. In truth, it can be freeing. That is what you want to feel, right?"

"Right."

"Benefit-cost time, Bob. Freedom-responsibility."

"Sounds like the obstacle part of the process."

"It is. The obstacle stage is important for a lot of reasons. It has several components. We won't specifically deal with some of the fears. I am not qualified to deal with those at any deep level. If you have any pathological fears, we'll send you to an expert. That kind of fear moves from obstacles into preparation. Going to a therapist becomes preparation instead of an obstacle."

"So how do you help me?"

"We'll try to figure out what obstacles you face in living your dream. Most of them will be small things that are recurrent, but not pathological. We can deal with those. Are you willing to try?"

"Yeah I think so."

"If it gets too scary, let me know. We'll go slow."

"Alright."

"Let's start with what I just told you about myself. What obstacles do you think I have faced?"

"Sounds like the biggest one is your adoption. It must be strange to not know much about who you are or where you came from. Have you ever tried to contact your parents?"

"Yes, about five years ago. The adoption agency found my mother. The law says the agency must contact the parents to see if they are interested in a reunion. After about six months I got a three-sentence letter from the agency. It just said they had contacted my mother. She wasn't interested in me. Didn't want to know anything. I pretended it didn't hurt for a while, but I couldn't hide it. It really hurt.

"One day they called out of the blue to tell me they had found my father. At first he denied being my father. After he met with the people at the agency, he finally admitted he was my birth father. He wrote to me and told me a little about himself. It was difficult. He was also going through a divorce. He was an alcoholic. It made me feel sorry he had been contacted. Imagine getting a call in the midst of a divorce and alcoholism that your 35 year-old son wants to meet you for the first time. His letters gave me some idea about him that I carry around with me. He wrote well, seemed articulate, and actually seemed to care. He seemed afraid.

"I wrote him once and told him about me, about my basketball career, about my position on the faculty at the medical school. He wrote back one more time. He told me about his relationship with my mother. He wanted me to know that I wasn't the product of a one-night stand. They had broken up when she told him she was pregnant. He figured I wasn't his, that maybe she had had another relationship. He said he just didn't want to accept it. He stayed with her through most of the pregnancy. In the early sixties, unmarried women went to benevolent homes during their pregnancies. He would visit and sit with her. Eventually it was too hard for both of them. Her parents were upset and just wanted it over with. They wanted him to disappear. So he left about a month before I was born. He never knew whether I was a boy or girl, or even if I existed."

"Wow. That sounds rough."

"I guess." He could see that I was struggling. My eyes fixed on the ground. I was fidgeting, my fingers moving constantly. "This is hard to talk about one-on-one. Sometimes when I give talks and I use terms that don't get through to the audience, I tell this story. There are usually two or three people in the audience who become tearful, who recognize the pain. They feel the same void of not knowing who they are, where they came from. They are reminded of it, every time they go to a doctor and have to give a medical history. They are reminded of it when they have to explain it to their own children. Many of them struggle in relationships, because they are looking for someone to prove to them that they are lovable. They want someone to forgive them, because they feel the first thing they ever did in life was to cause someone else pain."

He knew I was talking about myself. I knew it, too.

Obstacles

"So what do you do about that?" Bob asked.

"I needed to acknowledge that it was still affecting my life, that my behaviors were still responding to the belief that I was different, that I couldn't be loved.

"I grew up thinking I was reasonably in control of it. My parents had told me early that I was adopted. I can't remember not knowing. It was not until much later that I realized it was an obstacle for me, and I chose to do something about it. Benefit-cost. I didn't really know what the cost of dealing with it would be, but I knew it was getting in my way. In everything I have ever done I was pretty good, but I would always get to a certain level, and then the fear would show up as anger or a need for independence. I always had to do things on my own terms. It wasn't a control thing. I just needed to know that something could not be taken away from me. Maybe I felt like a fraud and was waiting to be found out."

"I know that feeling."

"So I took Dr. Davis's advice, and started learning from other people about how they got what they wanted in life. I learned a lot about people who had great lives and who had been through incredible emotional trauma. Nietzsche said, 'That which doesn't kill us makes us stronger.' I'm not sure that is true. Maybe the trauma can kill us in a way that we die so slowly, we don't even know it's happening. What I learned about these great people was that it was their response to the trauma that made the difference. They were all afraid, but it was how they responded to the fear that helped them grow."

"So what did you learn about yourself that applies to what you're teaching me?" asked Bob.

"I learned I was not alone in being afraid. That is why I was able to learn from people in such different areas of life. I can't play the piano or do surgery or swim. I hate dealing with money, so business would never to be a strong suit. When I listened and cut through all the cover language, I realized that my pain was not unique or deeper than most people's. I learned that the people who lived the way I wanted to all dealt with their own fear and problems. It was how they did it that was important."

"I got that feeling from talking to Jeff and to John," Bob said. "They both hit big obstacles that frightened them. Jeff losing in 1992 and John struggling with Hornsby to get their first record deal. Now that I think about it, Jeff must have been devastated when he lost in '92."

"Bruce talked to me about the anxiety of actually getting that first record deal," I told Bob. "He felt pressure to have a hit record and then a career. What's worse, the pressure they faced was front page. If they failed, it was public failure, and the press was waiting to rub it in. People knew who they were. I felt that in basketball. I sat on the bench on national television once a week. People at home never let me forget it. People in Charlottesville still talk to me about it 15 years later. Imagine what it would be like if everyday you had a newspaper reporter or television camera following you around at work, waiting for you make a mistake. Think what it would be like if your customers followed you around everyday and criticized every move you made with your boss standing right there."

"I can't even imagine. It's hard enough the way it is."

"There's a paradox in what I learned. While I knew I wasn't alone in my fear, I realized that people who haven't been adopted seldom understand how it feels. They struggle to imagine what it feels like not know to where you come from, what your heritage, what your medical history is. Many times when I talk to people about it, I can see them wondering why it hurts so much. I accept that they can't understand it, but that we can share our other fears and desires.

"Recently I read a book by a pro football player. He was adopted. He chronicled his experience, the nightmares when he was eight, the fear of being unlovable, and the effect on his relationships. Suddenly there was someone else who knew what I was feeling. He found his parents, but it cost him the people who raised him, his real parents. I decided when I read that, maybe the cost of finding my birth parents would be too high because of the effect it might have on the people I cared about and who cared about me. I have accepted that things have worked out for the best."

"I understand that."

"I went to a psychologist, a psychiatrist, a counselor. I tried all the conventional therapy I could stand. Only one thing in all that really helped me. After seeing the psychologist for a period, he confronted me. He said, 'Doug, you think this is going to cure you of the pain and the fear, don't you?' He was right. I thought that therapy would make things right, that I wouldn't have to deal with it again, if I just got help. He told me that I would never be cured of it. We were working towards an *acceptance* of the fear. His aim was to try to help me develop responses to the fear consistent with the rest of me.

"When the athlete wrote about the relationship between desire and fear, it clicked for me. I know there are fears that I am going to have. If I don't respond effectively, if I try to pretend I don't have them, or if I just hand my life over to the fear, I will never gain what I want in life. The cost of ignoring the fear or giving into it is just too high. I have to accommodate it in my life. That is why obstacles are part of the process. All of the people I interviewed knew that there would always be obstacles, and that sometimes they themselves created them. They tried to be a little better everyday. Some of the obstacles they could control, some of them they couldn't. What they taught me was that they could effectively respond to external obstacles and pursue the things they wanted in life. If the obstacle was an internal one such as fear or loneliness, they had to work out a response to their own response."

"Okay, now you're losing me."

"Do you have that napkin with you?" I asked.

"Sure." He pulled it out of his pocket.

Underneath obstacles I wrote:

External Obstacle-----Internal Obstacle-----Response to Response

"Let's go back to your life. Anything happen at work this week that you struggled with?"

"Yeah. Actually I was going to talk about it with you later. I screwed up something that cost the company some money. I lost a customer because we didn't quite understand his needs, and the solution we developed didn't solve his problem. In fact, it made things worse. My boss lit into me in a meeting. He didn't have to do that publicly. That's why I understood what you meant about Jeff and Bruce. About you sitting on the bench on national television. It wasn't national news, but it felt like it was, because the whole company seemed to know about it."

"When he was yelling at you, what was it like?"

"It was embarrassing. I felt some shame, felt like I wasn't good enough. I felt like a fraud. I beat myself up on the way home, even thought about quitting."

"Alright. So what was the external obstacle?"

"Well, I guess the first one was the mistake I made."

"Do you really believe that?"

"Sure what else could it be?"

"As I said earlier, we are going to make mistakes. We have to accept that. Suppose you had your own company, no bosses. You made this mistake and your customer calls and tells you about it. How would it be different?"

"I'd rush over, talk with the customer, and get clear on what they needed. I think the real problem was in the understanding of their needs. The solution we created solved the problem as I mistakenly saw it. I would do everything I could to make it right. In fact, I think I would enjoy that. I wouldn't like not getting it right, but I would do whatever it took to get it fixed and make the customer happy. If I owned my own business, I would do whatever it took to keep them happy."

"So the mistake actually wasn't the obstacle. It was more like a catalyst."

"Right. I see. I guess the obstacle was to know that there would be some evaluation of what happened, that I was going to be criticized, that there was some real risk of losing my job. When the boss publicly humiliated me, I got scared and started thinking I wasn't good enough."

"Right. The obstacle for you was the cost of the mistake and knowing there were consequences that you couldn't control. Whether it is true or not, the customer didn't seem to be as much of an obstacle as the people you work with. That was where the consequences really hit home. So he yelled at you publicly. That was the obstacle. But now that is over, right?"

"Well, not really. I'm still hurting over it. I'm still fearful of the outcome."

"Of course you are. But you still see being yelled at as the obstacle?"

"Yeah. Why?"

"Is he standing in here right now yelling at you?"

He laughed. "No."

"*Then the obstacle is now internal.* You are the obstacle. Your learned response, or even an innate response to being yelled at, is the obstacle."

"I get it."

"What can you do about it?"

"I've tried to put it out of my mind. That works some times, but it still creeps in every time I see him or am alone."

"Does that make things better?"

"It doesn't. It makes me doubt things I do. It makes me worry. I feel stupid, small, unaccepted."

Bob slouched as he talked. He felt the pain, reliving the moment.

Revisiting The Dream

"Do you want to make things better?"

"Of course."

"Are you willing to take some risks, to step up, and try again."

"Sure."

"Do you think you're good at what you do?"

"I did."

"Well, you haven't quit your job. You still get paid. You still show up everyday."

"Yeah."

"Then focus on the reasons you still do those things. Forgive yourself for making a mistake. What did you learn from this whole thing, not emotionally, but relative to how you do your job?"

"First, I had to be clear on what my customers want and need. I decided I had to have a closer relationship with my customers. My boss is always talking about having relationships with the customers. I guess this is what he was talking about. Secondly, we need to have a better way of dealing with the mistakes when they do happen so we can limit the damage."

"So focus on those things. Solve the problem. In order to solve the problem effectively, how do you need to feel about yourself and your skills? When do you perform the best?"

"When I am confident, when I am focused on the problem and my skills match it. No, that's not quite right. I guess when I feel I have some control over the outcome, either because I know that my skills are up to the task, or that I can learn enough in the time allotted to meet the demands of the task."

"So when you make a mistake with your customer, you feel you could work with him to do what it takes. And if you can't do what he wants, then the customer can see why it can't be done, or that it will cost too much money?"

"Right."

"So the obstacle is the relationship with your boss?"

"Sure."

"Can you control the relationship?"

"I don't feel like I have much control over it?"

"Have you tried to do anything about it?"

"Hide from him. Avoid him."

"And what does that do?"

"It makes the next time I see him more stressful. We communicate less. I'm scared to tell him anything in case he disagrees with me."

"Avoiding him, avoiding the fear, really makes things worse in the long run."

"Yeah , but it is easier."

"I told you this isn't easy. The question is whether or not it is worth the risk. Let's summarize. On one hand, you're scared of the boss and you avoid him, which makes you feel further out of the loop and worry more about losing your job."

"Right."

"The other option is to choose to learn from this, and to put strategies in place that might keep it from happening again. You need information from the boss to make changes. You need to do some homework. Build on what you know, and learn what you can to solve the problem. How do you think your boss will respond to you presenting a plan to fix similar problems in the future to make the customers more satisfied?"

"I hope he'll respond well."

"How do you want him to respond?"

"It'd be nice if he patted me on the back and gave me a few attaboys."

"Have you ever seen him do that?"

"No."

"So that's not reasonable to expect. Are the attaboys the only reason you want to do the work?"

"No, I want to be good at what I do. I don't like making mistakes, and I want to make it right."

"But the attaboys would be nice."

"Of course."

"You can't control that. The obstacle stage of things is about learning to control what you can, to hold onto what's right about you, and improve. My experience is that the obstacle stage provides the best opportunities to improve. It also sets you up to experience resonance, to engage in your life."

"How does it do that? I find that hard to believe. I would think they just cause pain."

"Remember what Jeff told you about the 1992 experience? He said that it was the best thing that ever happened to him. It was not so much the looking back at losing, but in realizing that swimming without Easy Speed and focusing only on the medal, were not the way he wanted to feel. He gained a deeper perspective. He hated the way it felt, and he was willing to do the work to feel better.

"That perspective didn't yet tell him how to solve the problem. If he didn't think about things, explore his pain, he would have merely trained harder, put in more laps, more time in the pool. He realized that it wasn't the amount of work he was doing, it was the way he was working. He felt pressure to win for the wrong reasons. He had to change the way he trained, the way he thought about swimming. He had to incorporate Easy Speed. It took him two years to figure that out.

"During that two years he kept working out, doing the technical work and training he needed to do, but he added a component to it. He dealt with the pressure. He realized that it was the perceived expectations of his family and friends that were adding to the pressure. He realized how the media felt about him, so he made a plan to respond to them. He learned from the 1992 experience. In doing so he took the obstacle away by moving it to the preparation stage. In 1996, he had a better idea of what he needed to do to alleviate the pressure.

"Your task is to learn from what happened, forgive yourself, and get back to work. Not just your job, but the work of creating the life you want, controlling what you can that matters."

"That sounds easy, but I'm sure it's hard to do."

"It is hard, especially the forgiving yourself part. You've already taken responsibility for what happened publicly, whether you wanted to or not. In some ways, that is a good thing that bosses do. They hold you accountable. What you do with that is up to you."

"Gotcha. That's scary, but it does make sense. Doing what I'm doing now certainly isn't getting me anywhere, and it certainly doesn't feel safe."

"The world is not a safe place. The only sense of safety you can have is to know that you can respond to the things that come up. You won't always get it right, and it won't always feel good. Not doing anything but retreating from your fear, not dealing with it, guarantees that you will not feel safe.

"There is a psychological concept called reactance. I juxtapose it with performance. The concept of reactance suggests that people will do anything they can to regain something that is taken from them. They'll fight like hell, even if the fight does more harm than good. In the long run, fighting is more costly, because it stifles growth, and prevents a person from reaching his or her potential. The fight becomes about what we have now, not what we can be. It keeps the focus on the past.

"Performance on the other hand is about the present and the future. Performers try to express an idea that they have created. They perform and then evaluate. How can I be better? They hold onto what is right about them and they set about being better; they improve. They still feel fear, they still grieve and mourn, but they don't get stuck in it. They have developed an internal process that allows them to look forward."

I pointed to the napkin again.

"Look at the obstacle stage. Follow the line clockwise. What's next?"

"Revisit the dream."

"Right. What I learned from the performers was that before they went and worked harder to fix something, they took time to see if what had occurred was genuinely an obstacle to their dream. In other words, had it really cost them, or was it a mere distraction? A lot of people hit an obstacle and go straight back to preparation. They work harder, but not smarter. In those cases, things that are actually irrelevant to their lives take up a lot of time and energy. If something important relative to their dream happens, they dive into the work even harder. Eventually they lose sight of why they are working so hard and burn out. When they get stuck between preparation and obstacles, they've lost their energy source, and they just work. I've had CEO's say to me that is when their people retire on the job."

"Boy, that sounds familiar. So how do you avoid that?"

"Well, you can't always avoid it. Everyone gets stuck there at one time or another. But if you keep track of why you are doing something, it makes it easier to hold onto. It's not just looking at this napkin. It has to be an active process. I call that Revisiting the Dream. When the feeling gets taken away, how do you get it back? How do you reengage in your life, the life you truly want?

"The first thing you do is find things, simple things, like songs, books, movies, places, activities that you know will remind you of the feelings you want, what you like about yourself. In a more passive sense, you surround yourself with people and things that automatically remind you of the good part of you. Some people would say that is avoidance, but not the way I mean.

"Obstacles are going to happen. They are a part of life. The trick is to acknowledge the obstacles, and have a plan to deal with them. Some of them will be external, but those are rarely the principal problem. They just set something off in each of us that creates an internal obstacle like fear. If you respond to the external with an appropriate short-term internal response, that's human. When your boss yelled at you, it hurt. It frightened you and you withdrew. We all do that. But if you stay withdrawn so you won't have to feel it again, you limit yourself. You'll never get to feel the way you want. Over time you just won't feel anything. Or you'll spend all your time trying to undo the past.

"That is one thing I face with the adoption issue. I try to make up for the loss of my mother by trying to convince someone I'm lovable. I can do that by responding to their needs. I'm good at that, but pretty soon I realize that I'm not getting what I need, because the other person doesn't really know me or what I need. There is no mutuality in the relationship. Then, sadly, it all blows up.

I have worked on myself to know what I need in life and how to get it. That is an ongoing process. I have to make observations. Believe me, I don't always get it right. I can tell you, though, the more I work on myself and the less I focus on just trying to be loved, the better my relationships are, and the more I actually have to offer other people.

"That is what Bruce was saying about 60% of his life being the 'baddest mother in music,' and the other 40% trying to get along with others. He knew he could not be alone and be happy. But if all he did was to try to give others what they wanted, he wouldn't create his own vision. He'd lose the desire and energy to make music. What a loss that would be. It's about finding what you want, what you're willing to work for, and then surrounding yourself with people in a way that mutuality can exist. It's a win, win situation."

"Wow. That sounds great."

"Yeah, but it takes work. That is why the revisit part is so important. You need to remember what you want, what you're willing to work for. If you fight too hard over something in the past, you are reacting and not growing. The revisiting allows you to grow and make more informed decisions about how to respond to things."

"I've got a story about the preparation-obstacle trap as you call it."

I was exhausted. I knew I couldn't listen to him effectively right now.

"Let's get together in two weeks. Save the story for that time. Is that alright?"

"Yeah. Two weeks." He seemed disappointed.

Responding To My Own Responses

When the pain hits me in the stomach, it buckles my knees and slightly paralyzes me. Sometimes it starts slow. If I pay attention, I can acknowledge it and welcome it as an old friend, a known adversary, as one psychologist taught me. Other times, it blindsides me. I feel it like raw emotional energy surging through my body right to the pit of my stomach. It's the physical loneliness, the lack of intimacy, the absence of another's touch.

As I sat out by the lake, under the blue sky dotted with small clouds, it hit quickly. I wasn't surprised. I had given a valediction speech the night before at a local high school. Sharing my message, connecting with others, especially high school kids, felt great. As soon as my talk was done, though, I was ushered out the back to beat the traffic, to drive home alone and vulnerable. This was the typical scenario that triggered feelings of inadequacy, reminding me that no one was waiting to share with. As I sat there, I knew these feelings actually signaled something different. I rarely doubt myself anymore. The feelings I had were more of a longing, of a wishing for more. They triggered old habits, old responses.

When I woke that morning, I had walked out to the lake, and plopped down on the shore. Boo and Raige followed through the tall grass taking time out to chase each other. Boo climbed onto my chest as I lay there. Raige moved cautiously, watching a beaver swim across the water with a stick in its mouth, one end sharpened like a spear. The beaver and his friends had ravaged the trees that rimmed the lake.

I felt Boo purring through my chest. Once again, I had done something fun and engaging, my talk, only to come home to be alone. That was when the pain hit. In the past, I would have found something else to do, to occupy my heart. Now I could sit still and let it surge through me like a seizure. It would end soon enough, and I wasn't going to let it ruin this moment by the lake. I felt myself breathe deeply, starting in my stomach, through my chest, and into my throat. I wiggled my toes and touched my fingertips against each other. When I tense up, when I am snowboarding, rollerblading, presenting, I judge my performance at some level by whether or not I can feel my fingers and toes. That was a way for me to know I was relaxed, that I was engaging all of me. I felt my fingers come to life and started to stroke Boo. She instantly rolled onto her back and off my chest playfully striking at my fingers. We wrestled for a few minutes, and just as suddenly as it had come, my emotional seizure was over.

This one piece of information was so important to me. I call it my response to my response. As a basketball player, an angry response to something in a game focused my attention, calling my physical abilities to bear on the task at hand. It was inner anger physically expressed by the demands of the game. Running harder, jumping higher, standing my ground, protecting the ball. As a teenager, in college, and for several years after, basketball had been the focus of my life; anger was my response to situations. In the short-term world of sport, it seemed to get me what I wanted. Many people saw me as an athlete, and they accepted this behavior as part of that identity.

I wondered what discovering the power of anger had cost me in life. I remember when I became aware of it in basketball. As a junior, I had a couple of bad games in a row and skipped practice to spend time with a girl. My coach was furious. He lit into me, telling me that he almost didn't start me. I got mad at him, because he just didn't understand how much I was beating myself up for the bad games, how mad I was at him for berating me.

A few nights later, we played the best team in our district. No one expected us to win. The game started slow and we hung in there. In the second quarter, I turned the ball over, and Coach chewed me out in front of the cheerleaders. I was embarrassed. I had a crush on one of them. I was furious.

In the next few minutes I scored twelve points, making several steals and several jumpers. They couldn't bring the ball up against me. At halftime, I collapsed in the locker room, exhausted. We won by a comfortable margin, but the lesson stuck with me: through anger, I could summon my physical prowess to do wonderful things. For the next ten years, I embraced that lesson.

As time passed, though, I wasn't getting what I so desperately wanted, connection to other people. The physical expression wasn't enough, because I didn't play. I had no responsible outlet. Words became my weapon. I would get to a certain level and get stuck, whether it was at work, in school, or in relationships. I knew I could do better, but I wasn't sure how. I was never violent or abusive, but I didn't walk away either.

The people I interviewed had hit major obstacles, both internal and external. Somehow they got past them. I found it hard to believe that they didn't have similar emotional responses to their experiences. They cared deeply and personally about the things they were doing, but somehow they were holding onto their dreams, improving, and eventually arriving at a place they could live their dream most days. They responded differently to similar feelings. My psychologist had implied it, when he told me to welcome my feelings of abandonment.

In essence, what all these people had said to me was this: You will have an innate or learned response to something you experience. Maybe that response is instinct or habit. Ultimately, what is important, though, is how you respond to your own response, before you respond to the obstacle itself. In simpler terms, it means get yourself together before you deal with the external situation. I describe it as my response to my response.

For most of my life, I simply responded. There were times when something angered me or hurt me. I knew I wouldn't be able to deal with the consequences if I reacted, so I squashed the response. In doing that, I didn't process the lesson, I wasn't learning about myself. I was simply giving in to the moment. I wasn't being myself. At the very least, I needed a way to learn from these interactions. Why was I angry? Why would something hurt me?

At other times, the consequences of responding weren't so apparent and I just reacted. Over time, I wasn't getting where I wanted to be. I had to look at my role in my own demise. I was the only common denominator in the equation. I must have been doing something wrong. I wasn't responding to my own response, before responding to the experience.

Boo curled up next to my arm. Raige meowed, rubbing against my hand looking for love. I thought about George Carlin, the comedian, whose routine included an observation about cats. He said that cats could do the dumbest thing like running into a plate glass sliding door, shake it off in a second, and then act like they meant to do it. He wondered if they then went behind the couch and said "Freaking Meow!" Cats were too cool for that. Boo and Raige didn't care what I thought about what they had done. If Jazz and Righteous do something stupid, like bite at a yellow jacket only to have it sting them, they come running to me just like little kids to their mothers. But cats have cool figured out. They just don't let it bother them. They move onto what's next in their lives.

In working with people, I have seen how important this lesson of responding to your response can be, how empowering it is, how freeing. For years, as a guy, I was told that I wasn't supposed to cry or to feel things. Boys learn how to respond to their responses by hiding them and filing them away never to deal with them. These lessons came from a variety of sources, but never from my parents. If I cried, they understood. The real pressure came from other guys.

Boys are taught a very limited range of emotions that are acceptable for us to have or to feel, much less to share. I can't count the number of men whose greatest source of shame is that they don't feel like a man, because they actually have emotions, though they still hide them. Maybe this is what Thoreau meant when he said that all men lead lives of quiet desperation. I decided I wasn't going to live that way.

I skipped some rocks across the pond, one skipping thirteen times. I felt the boyhood joy of my arm at play, manipulating the thin rock into a flat spinning motion. Boo and Raige watched with their feet on the water's edge. I thought about the fact that I feel younger at thirty-eight than I did at twenty-eight. My only guess is that anger and imposing power had aged me. Feeling trapped in solitude had disconnected me. If that's what being a guy is all about, you can have it.

Emotions are a crucial part of success and engagement. When I had surgery on my knees, one of the first things we did in rehab was to ensure a good range of physical motion. My response to my own life had to be to develop an emotional range that fit the life I led, the life I wanted.

Jazz and Righteous waited for me as I walked back to the house. I chased them around the yard, then fell to the ground and let them dig their noses under my head. I hoped Bob understood the response-to-response concept. That is what makes the dream part of our lives so important. The dream gives us a safe place, a foundation. The responses I want to have should engage me and help me get closer to living the dream. Having the dream, knowing how I want to feel each day, each moment, allows me to choose the response that gets me closer to that. Without knowing how we want to feel, how do we choose our responses? Too many people give up their dreams and live for safety. They please themselves largely by pleasing others. For me, that cost is too high.

Processing why I responded to certain situations so emotionally, I understood that I needed to know where those responses came from. Some were easy to figure out. My life as a baby taught me to brace against threats. Some of these feelings, the anger, the loneliness, the frustration, predated linguistic ability, preceded my internal dialogue. When my friends have had kids, I watch them in a crib or lying on the floor. They constantly wiggle their legs testing them out. I couldn't do that as a baby because of my surgeries and the plaster casts and braces holding them in place. Man, that must have driven me crazy. Understanding the effect of my adoption on my responses is a life-long challenge.

Some of my other responses, though, were learned from others. I have made an active effort to process those, to review my life, understand where I learned certain responses, and to recognize whom I learned them from. As a kid, I questioned authority probably more than most, but I challenged it responsibly. I was exposed to other people's ideas at a time when I wasn't free to express my own, or didn't know the freedom existed. I was still in training.

My responsibility as an adult is to stop responding to habit, and to choose the responses that fit me and connect me to the people around me. Exercising freedom in my life starts with discovering and freeing myself from what I think I know that may actually be irrelevant. I must learn from others and myself, and make sure that my responses are a choice, not simply habit or something I accepted as a child. Growing up, we don't have much choice about the person from whom we learn. As an adult, I can choose the people and the lessons I want to adapt to my life. I found and interviewed people on my own time. I made time in my life because it was important. It was what I would work for.

I decided to go rollerblading, so I jumped in the car and drove out to a local farm that was being developed into a subdivision. No houses had been erected yet, but the roads were newly paved with no traffic. Gentle rolling hills of the purest asphalt in town. On the outskirts of Charlottesville, old farms were being bought up by developers and turned into upper middle class neighborhoods. This was prime rollerblading real estate. No people, no cars, no bumps. I parked on the side of the road, threw on my blades, and searched for the simple rhythm of one foot pushing off after the other. My hands tucked into the small of my back, breathing from my stomach and up into my chest. Distant mountains surrounded my rural version of an asphalt playground.

Several weeks earlier, a young boy had walked into an elementary school out west and murdered his teachers and classmates. I don't know why that image popped into my head. I heard the song "Jeremy," by Pearl Jam, playing in my mind as I glided across the smooth pavement. The video ran in my mind's eye, a young boy shooting his classmates, the words, "Jeremy spoke in class today," playing in my ears. It bothered me that I understood why someone might do that.

I've told my parents that if it weren't for them, if I had grown up under different circumstances, there's a good chance I would be in jail. I'd been around kids who lived in the inner city. They went to the playgrounds to play ball, not because they had dreams of playing in the N.B.A., but for sanctuary. Several did end up in jail, and others ended up dead. Inside, they weren't much different than I, but their lives were far more limiting than mine was. I'd experienced the rage first hand in my trips to D.C., the threats, the fights, the guns.

Too many people think that violence and rage are just by-products of the inner city culture. My own experiences, though, told me otherwise. I felt similar feelings of disconnection. I had parents who saw what was going on in me, and did what they could for me. They didn't solve it, but they gave me healthier ways to respond. I had good schools, caring teachers, and helpful coaches. They were there to provide a lifeline. It added up to an implicit hope for the future. It was a hope many of my basketball friends never knew. I had choices.

When I see a homeless person on the street, or the guys with the signs that say they will work for food, I know that I could easily be one of them. I don't see the torn clothes or the disheveled appearance, as much as I see the pain and the humiliation. The guys I used to play ball with downtown seemed to have only the playground as a safe haven, as a place to express their creativity. As I've grown older, I've realized that so many feel the same things. It is their responses that make the difference.

As I glided along, another image ran through my head. It was of the time when I was in high school and part of a program that tutored kids in one of the most deprived neighborhoods in the country. I remembered waiting for Christopher, my student, in his kindergarten class, while he grabbed his books.

As I waited, another boy slapped the girl next to him, and then stood his ground ready for a fight. The little girl cried, and the teacher came running. "Antoine hit me," said the girl. I was shocked at what happened next. The teacher told Antoine to stand with his hands behind his back. Then she instructed the little girl to slap his face. The girl hesitated; Antoine's eyes grew big. "Hit him," demanded the teacher. The girl slapped Antoine across the face. His head jerked back, but he pulled it forward again defiantly, glaring at the teacher. The little girl cried. Antoine shook back his tears, not giving an inch. "Sit down, both of you," demanded the teacher. They both sat in silence, staring at their desks. It didn't make either one of them feel good. The teacher walked away triumphant, as though she had made a point.

I bladed down a slight hill, cutting back and forth. The secret to sports involving your feet such as blading, snowboarding, or even windsurfing is to gain back the energy you gave away, to feel the energy with your feet. When I can remember to pay attention, it is an tremendous feeling. Each push to the side with my feet generates energy back from the ground that travels up through my body. I share my energy with the ground.

I thought about how much that one moment had bothered me when I was tutoring. I remembered six-year old Christopher shaking his head as we walked into the hallway. "That was stupid," he said simply. It seemed Christopher, at six, already understood the response-to-response concept.

The experience stayed with me on several levels, but one was particularly disturbing. Hadn't I been taught similar lessons growing up by people around me? I was rewarded for being tough, for getting into fights on the basketball court, called a chicken if I didn't participate in bench-clearing brawls. I embraced that image, once described in the newspaper by an opposing coach as: "nasty, a real fighter." A Duke University student newspaper article called me, "a thug, the enforcer."

As I grew physically, the playgrounds changed. A fight used to be a fistfight. You stood your ground and didn't back down. You went hard into the opponent, stood over him when you knocked him down. Somewhere along the line, though, guns became part of the landscape. Once when I embarrassed an opposing player, he followed me to the parking lot and threatened me with his gun. Now on playgrounds in many neighborhoods, wealthy or poor, white or black, the first hint at being "dissed" leads to threats of "getting a cap in your ass." The threat carries weight because of the chance that someone might actually do it. I stopped playing on the playground a long time ago. There was something missing. The sanctuary was gone. Too many playgrounds now sit vacant.

I was pushing hard, bent over in a speed skater's position, long slow sweeps with my blades. I was sweating hard, recalling the one hundred plus degree heat of the playgrounds of summer. I shed my shirt and turned around in the cul-de-sac to head back over the two-mile road. I thought about how different I was now from that courtside brawler.

Response-to-response. Separating who I was from what I had been taught. Learning to choose, to exercise my freedom, to expand my range of responses. That is what I try to do now, though not always successfully. Jim Clawson, a friend of mine who teaches at UVa's Darden Business School, once wrote:

Unfortunately, many live their entire lives unsuccessfully seeking to fill their emotional holes by seeking attention from others. Many die never filling those holes or attaining the pervasive sense of power that accompanies it. The challenge is for each generation to keep from passing on its scars to the next generation.

Jim's words echo the commitment I have made so recently in my life. I will not pass on my own angst through poorly made choices. Ignorance and pain are no longer an option or an excuse. My choice is to free myself from myself, from my past, a past that was not always of my making.

I can only imagine the pain a mother goes through in giving up a child she has carried for nine months. It is a moment of physical and emotional separation, an indescribable trauma. The courage she must have shown. I think of my own birth mother, abandoned by the man with whom I was created, her parents embarrassed enough to warehouse her in a home, the shame she must have felt. She went through it for me, a powerful but hidden sign that I must matter, that I did count.

I curled around the end of the car, cranked the stereo, and sat on the bumper removing my blades. I thought about what it cost me, how traumatic my birthday still feels. I re-experienced the images of the recurrent nightmare my fears had created for me so vividly over the years:

I cried out as the nurse rushed me from the delivery room and into the long, sterile corridor. I longed for my mother, but I'd never see her again. I felt confused, lost, abandoned. Alone. They say babies know more than most people imagine. I knew I was a mistake.

My legs twisted, pointed in the wrong direction. I was no good. They would have to fix me. Nobody would want me this way. She certainly didn't want me.

The nurse wrapped me in the blue, coarse blanket. My small crib was cramped into the back corner of the large, dimly lit room. Babies cried all around me. Men pressed their smiles against the window while pointing at other babies. No one pointed at me. Other babies were taken away. New babies took their places.

They fed me, changed my diapers, and then dumped me back in my crib. The cloth masks hid their faces. Their touch was shielded by latex.

They never held me long. I wanted contact, the touch of another's warm skin. I'd cry out. Nothing. Something was desperately wrong. I knew it. My legs hurt all the time. I was afraid.

Weeks later, the nurses returned me to the room where I had last felt my mother. I saw the same masked faces, felt the same rubber-gloved hands. As I neared the table, my body readied for the touch of my mother. I felt the excitement growing, the warm feeling of being wanted, of being loved, of the womb.

I suddenly felt threatened. There was no one on this table. My body stiffened. I instinctively held my breath. The bright lights hurt my eyes as I was placed on the table. They stuck me with needles. They painted my legs a messed-up orange-yellow color. What was happening? Where was my mother? Didn't she care? Didn't anyone care?

I fell asleep, angry and scared. Sleep changed forever that day. Hours later, I awoke with heavy plaster on both legs. When I moved, I felt the pain of my scars rubbing against the casts. Yet the physical pain offered escape from the wrenching betrayal and isolation of being ignored. Physical discomfort and darkness became my friends. Such friendship was my only recourse.

The instincts of this small boy, this infant--despite the darkness and the pain--demanded survival.

If my fear, my pain, was so strong, so vivid, what must hers have been like? I knew my response to rejection, to failure, to success might always be the pain in my stomach. I owed it to her to have the courage, the knowledge, to respond wisely to it. I owed it to her to broaden my choices, to expand my range of options, in responding to the pain and fear.

Moving past my own response, moving beyond the feelings of self-pity, became freedom for me, and the fulfillment of my responsibility to her. She must have believed in me to thrust me into the world as an illegitimate child. It was why she had been strong enough to carry me to term. I wouldn't dishonor her courage, her strength, her love, by giving into the same fear she faced so gracefully, so effectively.

My response to my response is to choose for myself, to pass along hope and life, and not impose my fear on those around me. That is the intimacy she and I share: fear diminished by desire, love overcoming pain. By loving myself, by living my dream, I love and honor her. In my mind, she is one of the unvanquished, living a life beyond simple survival and selfishness. Her later rejection does not change that.

My Jeep rolled through the winding mountain roads and back towards Buck Mountain, back home. For the first time in my life, I'd allowed myself to think consciously and explicitly about what she'd been through, what she'd done for me. The insights of others, my friends and those I interviewed, had helped me to see beyond my selfishness, past the fear inside of me. The feelings of inner freedom overwhelmed me, excited me.

Doubt still lived, old habits died hard, but the recognition, the acknowledgement, of what she'd done for me freed me from the belief that the first thing I'd ever done in life was to devastate someone else's life. The intimacy of this day, the intimacy of one body growing inside another, gave birth to an empathy for her sacrifice and a new found freedom for me.

Chapter 7

The Ability To Be Alone

Disconnected, Not Independent

Bob and I had agreed to meet at the local Barnes & Noble bookstore. I went there everyday to read the newspaper. I always paid for the papers, but left them there for others. It was a simple way of making my life easier. No more piles of papers at the house to mess with.

Bob was seated in the corner slowly turning his coffee cup around a half turn at a time. He stared down through the cup, who knows where, as the rhythmic motion of the turning cup mesmerized him. I slid onto the hard wooden bench, turned sideways and put my feet up. He barely noticed me.

"What's going on?" I said to him.

Without looking up, he kept spinning the cup slowly with his thumb and forefinger. "I don't know," he whispered.

Uh-oh, I thought. He was struggling with something. I wondered when this would happen. People look at the process and think it is easy, because it is simple. It is difficult to do and to maintain over any extended period of time. It is an active process. It takes exercise.

"At the risk of a cliché, what are you feeling?"

"Alone."

"Can you be more specific? What other feelings do you have?"

"Scared. Empty. Disconnected." He looked up for the first time. His eyes were hard, but sad. He was relaxed, though. There was an absence of tension in him, which surprised me. He seemed to know that these feelings were real. Real was alright. He had made a lot of progress since I first met him.

"What are you afraid of?"

"People don't understand what I'm doing. They think I'm being childish. Several people at work have told me that I just need to be strong, to buckle down and get on with my life."

"Why did they tell you that?"

"I guess because I have tried to share with people what I've learned, what I've experienced. They just don't get it. They understand what I'm trying to achieve, but they don't think the process will work."

"Do these people who are telling you this live the way you want to live?"

"No."

"Then why are you listening to them?"

"I guess because they are the closest thing I have to friends. Maybe that's what this is about. I don't feel as though I have any real friends."

"Why do you think that?"

"I never really thought much about friendship. I just took for granted that the people in my life were my friends because I worked with them and they had some similar experiences with me. You know, we all know what work is like. We can empathize with each other."

"So you can sit around and complain about things."

"I guess so. Man. That doesn't sound very fulfilling. That's accurate, though. If I think about it, that is what our relationships are."

"When you do that how does it make you feel?"

"Angry, but connected. I don't feel alone then. When we sit and talk about all the lousy things at work, we get all wound up. It does give me energy."

"Do you ever do anything about the problems?"

"No." He looked up again. The anger swept through him. Now he was tense. "We just hunker down and become like warriors who are trying to win some battle. The war never seems to end, though. Our conversations merely become a way to steel us for the next fight. I'm tired of fighting."

"What do you want to do about it?"

"Well, coming to you was the first step for me. Look, I think I understand what you've been showing me. I must admit, though, I'm uncomfortable. The more I know about myself and about what I want in my life, the more I feel like I am disconnecting from the people around me. Then I start feeling alone."

"You mean you feel lonely?"

"Yeah, same thing."

"Actually it's not. Remember what you told me the first time we met, that you wanted to be free to do things for yourself, for your own reasons. Well, that requires being alone sometimes. You might need to be alone to think, to re-energize, to do things that others don't want to do. Actually, being alone is the best way to understand what really matters to you in life, to identify what's important and what you will work for."

"How so?"

"Think about your life. How many times have you compromised your own values, or accepted some responsibility, just so you would be liked or so you could be part of something? Probably very often. The more you do that without being alone, the more likely it is that you forget who you are, what you want. Learning to be alone is important."

"But it's really frightening."

"I know, but being frightened is real. The question is how can you be alone and deal with that fear?"

"I don't know. That sounds hard."

"It is. So ask yourself if you're willing to do the work, to learn to be alone."

Bob seemed uncomfortable. He hitched his belt, running his fingers along the inner edge of his pants. Though he said he wanted to do something for himself. He was probably afraid of being alone with his thoughts, with silence. Psycho-analyst Donald Winnicott once wrote that, "More has been written on the fear of being alone or the wish to be alone than on the ability to be alone...it would seem to me that a discussion on the positive aspects of the capacity to be alone is long overdue." It was time to have this discussion with Bob

A Trip To The City

"So I just forget my friends, my family?"

"Not at all. What I'm saying is: know what you want, so you can help others help you. Being alone is an important part of that. Being alone, dealing with the fear, can show you strengths you didn't know you had. If I dropped you in a big city for a week where you didn't know anybody, what would you do?"

"I'd feel pretty scared and alone."

"I didn't ask how you'd feel. I asked you what you'd do."

He started turning the cup again. His eyes closed. He seemed to stiffen at first and then slowly loosened up. He was solving the problem. He engaged himself.

"I think, initially, I wouldn't do anything. I would just give into the fear. That would paralyze me. If I knew I had to stay for a week, though, I would first figure out where I was going to stay. I'd probably check into a hotel."

"A nice hotel or a dive?"

"Nothing extravagant. I would just want be comfortable."

"Then what?"

"I'd probably hang out there for a while, watch some television."

"Why?"

"Again to feel comfortable, to take my mind off being alone."

"But you're still alone?"

"Yeah. I guess what I'm saying is that I would familiarize myself with the surroundings. I'd make it safe for myself."

"Exactly. Then what?"

"I'd probably go down to the desk and ask about things to do, places to eat."

"What do you think the desk manager would ask you?"

"I don't know what you're asking."

"Well, my experience with hotel management people is that they will ask you what you like to do, what kind of food you like. Then they'll make suggestions. Then you have to choose."

Okay. I'd tell him I like going to the movies and I want a nice juicy steak."

"Suppose you choose to go to a movie. How do you feel going to a movie by yourself or eating in a restaurant by your self?"

"I thought about that. I think my first meal, I would order room service and just check out the pay-per-view in the room."

"So why wouldn't you do that all week?"

"I'd go crazy. I'd probably get bored. I would probably be on the phone to my family and to my wife. Maybe a couple of friends."

"Stay with that for a second. How would you decide who to call?"

"I'd call my family, because they would care about me. They would want to know how I was doing, and I would wonder how they were doing."

"Is that all? What would you feel if you talked to them?"

"I don't know. I wouldn't feel so alone. I'd remember that there was someone out there who cared. I think I would also stop thinking about myself for a while, because I'd be concerned about them. I suppose I would feel connected to someone."

Even though I was sitting right in front of him, Bob was afraid. His mind drifted off. He was imagining himself sitting in his hotel room alone. He looked like a lost little kid.

My mind raced to a dream I used to have. In the dream, I was that lost little kid running from door to door on a dark, dismal street. A single streetlight created shadows by the buildings. It was right out of Dickens. I would knock on doors, crying for help. The night air enveloped me in a dreary mist. Families darkly shadowed their windows, pretending not to see me or to let me in. The little children were laughing at me. My guess was that Bob was seeing similar images in his mind, alone in that hotel room.

Friendship

"What about your friends. Who would you call?"

"I have to think about that. I know if I called the people at work, it would just be about how lucky I was to be away. I'd worry about my job. I don't think I'd call someone at work."

"So who would you call?"

He looked sad again. He just sat there. His shoulders slumped.

"What are you thinking?" I asked him.

"I was thinking that if I could call anybody in the world, I would call my brother and maybe some friends from school. I have stayed in touch with a few guys from school, from my fraternity."

"Why would call them?"

Bob sat silent for a while. He cocked his head away from me. He seemed ashamed. I put my hand on his forearm and stayed quiet.

"I'm picturing myself being in this city, in this hotel room, cable on, food tray next to me on the bed. It actually feels pretty good."

"Then why do you seem so sad?"

"Because I realize what I lost over the past 15 years."

"What's that?"

He looked me in the eye again. "Myself, parts of me that I liked. The curiosity. Seeing life as an adventure, my adventure. Being in that city, in that hotel would have been exciting when I was twenty. I'd have wanted to learn as much about the city as I could. I'd have stayed out at night. I'd have had fun."

"What made you realize that?"

"What you asked me about who I'd call. I realized I wouldn't want to call the people I'm around most of the time, other than my family. I guess I would see this as an opportunity, once I was comfortable with the place. I'm ashamed that I felt lonely and scared at first. I know if someone else said that to me, I'd laugh at them and just tell them to relax, even though I didn't do it myself." He let out a sarcastic laugh.

"So being alone, feeling lonely, would lead you to do something about it. You'd take care of yourself first. You'd make yourself comfortable in your surroundings, and then connect with people who made things better yet. By being alone, you reintroduced yourself to a part of you that you'd forgotten. Why did you do that?"

"I guess I felt that was the only choice I had. If I stayed paralyzed, I would have been at risk. I mean I wasn't going to sleep in the street, or even in a dirty hotel. I wanted to feel safe."

"So you took some action. You sized up the situation, and made choices based on what you wanted, not just on what you needed."

"What do you mean?"

"Well, you didn't go to just any hotel because you needed shelter. You made a conscious decision about how you wanted to feel. Then you went beyond that and said, 'What do I want?' You chose a restaurant or room service based on what you wanted. You went to a movie, because the cost of feeling alone at the movie was a better feeling than sitting alone in your hotel. I go to movies by myself a lot. People give me a hard time about that. They always tell me they could never do that because of what others would think, or that it would remind them they are alone.

"When I got divorced I had a choice to make. Either I could only go to movies that my friends wanted to see, and when they could see them, or I could go see the movies I wanted to, when I wanted to, but alone. It was the same with going out to eat. I mean we're not talking about things you plan weeks in advance. I wanted the freedom to go out to eat, or to go to a movie when I wanted to go, on the spur of the moment. That is hard to do with busy friends.

"The lesson of all this is that the freedom I needed was not from other people, but from my own fear. Pretty soon I got to the point where I enjoyed going to movies by myself, because my schedule allows me to go in the afternoon when it's cheaper and less crowded. When a movie comes out that everyone is talking about, I can go without worrying about crowds."

"But don't you worry about what other people think?"

"I used to, but I forced myself to go, because once the theater went dark, everyone was into the movie. Eventually, I enjoyed it and the fears of what others might think went away. The bottom line, though, was that I wasn't going to let what others thought control my life. The cost of not doing that was too high for me. Then I started seeing benefits that I hadn't thought about, like cheaper tickets and smaller crowds. I found that I enjoyed the movies even more. If there is a movie I want to share with someone I can still go with them, when they can go."

"I get it. Boy, that seems so simple, but it is still scary."

"Remember benefit-cost. Even freedom from yourself costs something. Let's get back to the discussion about your friends. Tell me about your friends from school. Why did you want to call them?"

"I'd call them because they remember the parts of myself that I really liked. When I talk to them there is an understanding. They've seen me at my worst and at my best. They know what bothers me and what I love. They didn't judge me the way people do now."

"Why do you think that is?"

"I have no idea."

"That's not good enough. Let's turn the question around. Why wouldn't you call people who are in your life now?"

That's easy. They don't know me. The part of me that I would feel in that hotel isn't related to work or even to my family."

"Let me take a guess. The Bob who is sitting in that hotel isn't defining his relationships merely by his responsibilities."

"What do you mean?"

"When you call your old friends, you don't owe them anything. They don't expect anything from you other than for you to be yourself, both the good part of you and the parts you like less. They are just your friends for better or for worse. You trust their opinions, because they can be honest with you. They can be right on the mark with you, because they know all of you. Other people expect something from you. You have measurable responsibilities in those relationships. You focus on living up to those responsibilities. The more you do that the more your freedom is threatened. That takes its toll."

"So again we're back to chucking all responsibilities."

"Not at all. Remember everything is a balance, a continuum between freedom and responsibility, between benefit and cost. We're not going to have a perfect balance in every relationship. The question is whether or not we can have balance across our lives. My friends give me a sense of freedom, when something in my life requires too much responsibility. If something goes wrong at work or, even worse, when I screw up at work, they are there for me to talk to about it. They help me gain perspective. They remind me how much they care. The most important thing they do for me is to keep me from taking on too much responsibility.

"The danger to me in what I do is that I can get too invested in the people I work with. Their problems become my problems. I feel everything. That can be draining. My old friends help me work through how to keep that from happening. They do that without judging me. I hope they feel I do the same for them. My friends also enjoy many of the same things I do, such as snowboarding, rollerblading, or just getting together to have thoughtful conversations about life. Knowing they are there gives me a sense of safety inside myself.

"Some of this may sound paradoxical in that learning to be alone also has improved my ability to be friends with people. I've learned to dig deep, to try as best I can to be honest with myself. Only then can I be truly honest with my friends. They know me. When they call me, they know I will be honest with them. I can only do that because I try to be honest with myself. I try to live what's inside of me. Learning to be alone, allowed me to discover parts of me that, in a crunch, I knew I could rely on. Although I am very good at being alone, I can't imagine my life without my friends."

"I think I just told you that I don't feel I have those kind of friends."

"Maybe you don't. I can't say. But you did say there were some people you would call when you were in a pinch. Aren't those your friends?"

"But we haven't stayed in touch as much as I would like to."

"So do something about that. Reach out to them. Plan things with them. When I went to my 20th-year high school reunion, I realized how little the part of me I liked had changed. My friends from high school and I acted just as we did 20 years ago, even though I had rarely talked with them. The nice thing in my life is that I have friends who make me feel that way now. They are spread all over the world, but I talk to one or another of them for a while almost every night. The most important thing is that I know all of them are there for me, and they know I would reach out for them. They know that about me, because I have been honest with myself about what's important to me. Friends head the list."

"That sounds awe-inspiring."

"It is. Believe me, it didn't happen just because I'm a good guy. I invested in each relationship. I am honest with them, and they are honest with me. If I ask them to lend me money, or to go give talk with me for free, or to listen to me when I'm hurting, they don't complain. Jeff Rouse and I have taken several trips together that haven't gone as planned. Long delays, running out of money, lousy hotels. We even joke about how something will always go wrong when we are together. But by being together, we always have fun.

"That happens because we decided that the friendship is important. We protect it. It takes work, but it rarely feels like work and it never involves a decision. The decision was made long ago that sharing our lives was important. I am a hard person to be friends with, because I don't tell people what they want to hear. I tell them what I think. The bottom line is that my friends trust me to be honest, and that I genuinely care about them.

"It took some work and some real risk on my part to show my parents who I am and what was important to me, but my parents are now my best friends. We struggled for a while, but we got there. They were great role models for me, because they have had great friendships with people lasting thirty and forty years. I can see how important those friendships are to their lives, and to how they want to feel about their lives. When they retired, they had a group of friends with whom they now travel all over the world. Best of all, they are good friends themselves. It comes back to the question, what are you willing to work for? If having a few genuine friends is important to you, what will you do to make that happen?"

"I could start by getting to know my friends from school again and letting them get to know me again"

"Sure, but remember to start by getting to know yourself at the same time. I work with a fair number of people. One common theme is that their life was darkest when they felt they didn't have friends. Almost every one of them changed that by getting reacquainted with themselves, so that they could choose their friends for good reasons. They learned that even when they were alone, they could enjoy their own company, and that having friends made their lives better.

"Friendship is more than just filling holes. If a person fills a hole in your life, it is easy to take them for granted and to neglect them. Then the relationship withers. It doesn't happen because we're bad people. It happens because the relationship is not stimulating enough in either direction. When you build a house, you start with the foundation, but then you spend most of your life in the living room or family room. If you don't check the basement enough, it can get moldy, cracks might develop, and it might even have serious leaks. Over time, the foundation needs major care.

"Your friends cannot serve as your foundation. Only you can do that. If you don't take care of it, of yourself, soon all you will have is an unsound superstructure that's no good to anyone. So start by visiting your basement, making the repairs, and strengthening it. Minor cover-ups won't do. What the rest of the house looks like, how it works, is limited by the shape and strength of the foundation. The great thing about friends is that they can help you discover rooms you have not yet enjoyed. But they, too, want to know that foundation is solid."

"Gotcha." He was sitting up and his hands had finally let go of the cup.

"So what's next?"

"I'm going to go think more about that week in the city. I'm going to imagine that I am there for the whole week, and see what I would do and why. It crossed my mind that after a few days, I would probably invite my friends or my family to join me for the remaining days. I hope I would do that, because it would make the trip more interesting, and not just to keep me from being lonely. Following that action might take a while, though."

"Sounds good. I'll see you next week."

Chapter 8

Remember And Forgive

It's More Than Talent

The phone rang at about 11:00 pm. It was Bob. His brother was having heart problems, and he wanted to know if someone at UVa. could see him.

"Sure, you should call Curt Tribble. He's my boss and best friend. I trust him with my life." I gave Bob his office number, and I paged Curt to tell him that Bob would be calling his office the next day. I knew Curt was either in the OR, doing paperwork, or working out. Curt and I sleep only a few hours a night. The time of day really means little to us. Sleep is to re-energize when we need it. Our emails often clock in at 4 am to each other. The difference between us is that Curt needs eighteen hours in a day just to get his work done.

It is ironic that Bob called when he did, because I was going to send Bob to see Curt at some point anyway. Not for his heart. Well I take that back. Not for his *physical* heart. I had learned as much from Curt as from anyone about how to apply the process in real life. Even though he works 100 hours or more a week, Curt also has an incredible appetite for life. He confronts life and death decisions and consequences every day. He can't afford to dwell too much on the obstacles in life. He also cannot afford to squelch emotional responses to crises. He has spent hours developing ways to apply lessons I now teach.

I met Curt at the hospital the next day. He had seen Bob's brother, Dave, and met Bob. They agreed to sit down and talk later that day. Curt had ordered an arteriogram on Dave, and was awaiting the results. He suspected Dave would need surgery, probably a CABG (Coronary Arterial Bypass Graft). They called it a cabbage. I also knew that before doing the operation, Curt would talk to Dave about the process. I asked Curt if Bob could sit in on this discussion. He said that was fine.

A week later Bob came to see me as scheduled.

"How's Dave?" I asked, even though I knew the answer. I wanted to talk about his brother and what Curt had done.

"He's doing fine. Dr. Tribble really fixed him up. That was nerve-wracking for all of us. Made me wonder. Dave's only a few years older than me. But he's not quite in the good shape that I'm in." He wrapped his hands around his middle and laughed. He was telling the truth, though. Dave was rotund.

"That 's good. How are you doing?"

"I'm good. What happened with Dave accelerated the process for me. I got scared and wondered what the hell I had done with my life. Dr. Tribble invited me in to listen as he and Dave discussed the surgery. It really surprised me when he asked Dave why he was in the hospital. Dave said there was something wrong with his heart. Dr. Tribble..."

"Call him Curt. It sounds too formal to hear Dr. Tribble. He would tell you that Dr. Tribble is his father."

"Yes, he did seem kind of young to be doing this stuff. How old is he anyway?"

"45."

"Really? He looked even younger than that. Anyway, Curt told Dave that's not what he meant. He wanted to know what Dave wanted to do with his life when he was better. What would he really miss if he couldn't do it? Dave had to think a while. This all sounded familiar. Dave said he'd play hoops with his kids and go dancing with his wife. Curt told him that throughout this process he wanted Dave to focus on that. It seemed to lighten Dave's worries. In fact, after Curt left, Dave couldn't stop talking about the last time he and his wife went dancing. He really is in love with her. I guess they don't get much time to go dancing anymore, or to even be alone. Curt asked Dave to send him a picture of him with his kids or dancing with his wife."

"Curt does that with many of his patients. Instead of focusing on the heart problem, it gives them something to look forward to, something to give them energy going through a rehab program."

"Yeah, that's "revisit the dream," right?"

"Yep. Did you get to spend time with Curt?"

"Sure did. We had a good talk. He really seems to care about helping people. Anyway, he told me all about his life, how he became a doctor, and how he is constantly trying to improve. I can't imagine what being a heart surgeon must be like. Man, these guys you've introduced me to all seem like regular people, but they do some amazing things."

"That's the point. If they were incredibly different, I would never send you to see them. They would just make you feel bad. I learned a lot from them, and the others I've interviewed, about how to be a normal person, but still to live an extraordinary life. At some level, it is talent. Equally important is that they lived in a way that allowed them to find their talent and to maximize it. That's all I'm trying to do with you. They just have a head start."

"But they seem so successful."

The Mickey Rourke quote about how painful his life was popped into my head again. The public perception that somehow talent and fame always make people happy is flat out wrong. People who are successful have a different set of problems, but they have just as many and just as difficult.

"Well, that's because you weren't around them when they were going through the tough times. I have a hard time convincing people that these leaders are not that different. There could easily be something that you are very talented at, but you haven't discovered it yet. It could be something you do right now, but that you still have to commit to finding and maximizing. That takes patience and work.

"Think about things you resonated with as a kid. You probably didn't love basketball the first time you tried it, but you wanted to learn about it. As you improved, you connected to it. That's why it's important to ask yourself not just what you want, but also what you will work for. Jeff, Curt, and John all worked an incredible number of hours to get better at what they do, but they also tried other things along the way to make sure that what they were doing was what they wanted to do. They did it with patience and without any guarantee they would be successful in a material sense. Their focus was different. Each of them had a vision inside of them of the way things could be. And they invested in themselves, in their skills, and in their passion to stay the course. How many people can you say that about?"

"Not many. They seem so confident, though. I don't think I have that kind of confidence."

"Maybe you do, maybe you don't. Let me tell you how I view confidence. There seems to be two perspectives on confidence. One is the media version of confidence. The way it is described on television, as far as I'm concerned, is dangerous. If I accepted it, I would assume that people like John, Curt, and Jeff never get nervous. I would think Dawn Staley believes that everything is always going to go the way she wants it to. That kind of thinking only distances us from their humanity. We say to ourselves exactly what you just said, 'I'm not that confident, so I won't try.' That creates a gulf between them and us. As a result people think they can never apply anything they learned from the example set by people like Dawn

"As a result of my conversations with them, I developed a more pragmatic view of confidence. Confidence plays a role in performance. If your view of confidence isn't useful in your performance, in your life, then why bother with it? The idea that confidence is the difference between success and failure makes it impossible for me to feel good about taking risks, about trying to perform at a higher level. That other view of confidence implies that if you don't have total belief that you will succeed, why would you ever try? If confidence is the main ingredient in success, how can people attempt the next level, knowing they have yet to succeed at that level?

"The way I see confidence goes back to the process we've been talking about. The question you must ask is, 'Is what you are trying to do worth the risk of potentially not succeeding?' My answer for many activities would be that it is definitely worth it, and that's an answer that let's you try. Here's why.

"First, I learned that all of these people faced obstacles, things you and I might think were show stoppers, like Jeff losing in 1992. If it were you and I, we might just quit. But these performers gave the obstacles they faced, including their failures, a meaningful role and that role is education. They created a lifestyle where they knew they could learn from obstacles. They surrounded themselves with people who still believed in them as people, even if they weren't successful at every attempt. They stayed in touch with their own visions of their lives and stayed true to it. While they were on the path, they didn't just chuck everything else and live irresponsibly. They compared their freedom to create their own lives against the responsibility they had to other people.

"Their confidence came from having a clear idea in their head of what they wanted to pursue. They made choices to pursue those ideas. They chose the people they wanted in their lives. Their confidence also came from some small initial successes. But it was the fact that they survived the rocky times, that later gave them a sense of confidence, of safety. A lot of people think confidence comes from success. I think it can also come from failing, trying again, and learning from that experience."

"Curt talked a lot about his patients," Bob reflected. "He said he looks upon each operation as a chance to learn something for future patients, as well as to help the current one. He knows he can't save everyone, but knowing that what he learns will help his future patients makes the difficult cases easier to deal with. He called it collective advocacy. I think what he means by that is that if something goes wrong, he owes it to his patients to learn from it. He can't afford to beat himself up during lunch, because a surgery he performed that morning may have had a difficult outcome. After all, he might have to do the same operation in the afternoon on someone else."

"Right," I answered. "Suppose Curt had had a grueling and ultimately unsuccessful surgery the morning before your brother's surgery. Would you have wanted him to walk in still doubting himself, still berating himself in the afternoon because something went wrong in the morning? Or would you have wanted him to learn something from the morning operation and come back into the OR ready to go to work on your brother?"

"That's a stupid question."

"But it is a question that is answered wrong every day by millions of people. The message we learn from too many coaches, parents, teachers, and bosses is that if we don't show disappointment, if we don't beat ourselves up, then we don't care. I'm not saying there shouldn't be some disappointment, but it should be measured and become part of the overall procedure. We need to incorporate the disappointment into our performance. Disappointment is inevitable in life, especially if you are shooting for the stars. The trick is to keep from getting mired in it.

"Too many people stop shooting for the stars, because they can't deal with past disappointments. They never let go. One reason is that we reward people who act accountable and say, 'It's my fault.' There is a sense of honor in it. But if they don't let go of it, day after day they set themselves up to make the same mistakes. They haven't learned anything, and they think it is enough to say they care, and they are sorry. They're not bad people. They just haven't learned how to deal with disappointment in an effective way. The best way that I've learned is what Curt talks about.

"Curt had always struggled against being a surgeon who talks about failures or bad results. Who wants to go to a surgeon who is an expert on failure? In working on this program, we thought long and hard about a way of dealing with poor performances, without being seen as poor performers themselves. The reality is that in every performer's life, poor performances happen. It is part of life. You can't ignore that part of it. We agreed to call them sub-optimal outcomes." It's not a "used car," it's a "previously owned car."

Sub-Optimal Outcomes

"Remember and forgive?"

"Right. So the best place to start is to learn from people who deal with disappointment well, who understand that it is part of the process. Do you think you have learned an effective way of dealing with mistakes and with failures?"

"I never thought about it before. I usually batter myself pretty good. Wow. What happens then is that I try to do exactly what someone else wants, so I won't disappoint him or her again, or I won't get yelled at anymore. Pretty soon, I feel bad because I am just living the life they want me to live. You called that reactance, I think."

"When you hit an obstacle and feel disappointment, it's natural to experience a let down. In your life, it might have a slow-drip effect over time. But for Jeff, Curt, and John, the timetable is much shorter. If Curt wallows in that "let-down" stage, he puts people's lives at risk. If John does that, he lets down his audience. If he puts on a bad show in Washington, D.C., he has to be ready to go to New York City and perform the next night. He has to get on a bus with the other band members after the show in D.C. and drive for 5 hours, get into the hotel late, and get up the next day and do it all over again. The band depends on Molo for tempo during the show. They all key on him.

"When Jeff lost in '92, he was demolished; he sat around getting down on himself for losing. He was embarrassed and didn't want to race in the relay the next day. He felt lost almost until the moment the race started. Team member, Pablo Morales came up to him in the ready room right before the race. He told him to forget about the night before and to go out and swim. Pablo said, 'We still care about you. Now go out and swim like you know how to.' Jeff learned something important with Pablo's help, despite the stress he was under. He realized that the night before he had put too much emphasis on the medal and not on the swimming. He'd forgotten about Easy Speed. Jeff knew he could go out and swim, and although he was physically depleted from the race the night before, he broke his own world record.

"If he had not listened to Pablo, if he had continued to berate himself, he never would have been able to do that. They needed Jeff to swim a great race, because the Americans had never lost the medley race in international competition, and the Russian team was very strong that year. If Pablo had said to him 'Hey you screwed up last night. We can't lose this race. You better swim well,' do you think that would have had the same effect?"

"No," Bob answered.

"But that was what Jeff was doing to himself. Pablo took him out of that, because he knew Jeff from training with him. What happens when you make a mistake at work?"

"Like I said, I get down on myself, mope around for a while, and just try to please everybody."

"Do you perform better?"

"No, I just stop performing period. I mean I get my work done, but not with any effectiveness or efficiency. Sometimes getting yelled at shakes me up, and I use that energy to achieve something, but it never lasts and I eventually get angry. Then I start blaming other people, even when it is not their fault.

"Obstacles are great educational tools, but only if they are dealt with effectively. I can't give you a formula for how to deal with them. What I've tried to do is give you a different perspective. I've also tried to show you that everybody hits obstacles, no matter how talented they are. All those guys talked about how much the obstacles meant for them in their development.

"Bruce Hornsby, the musician, said that at one point he had the producer, David Geffen, listen to him and say, 'Brucie, I want to make records with you.' He said he was jacked. Then Geffen signed John Lennon the next day and Bruce dropped down the priority list. He was really disappointed. Bruce tried to work something out with Geffen's company, but eventually they told him he wasn't ready, but to keep working, to keep getting better. Bruce was a bit offended, but he reflected on what they said. He went and got better. He didn't just beat himself up. He told me that they were right, that he wasn't ready, and thank God they didn't sign him. He might not have reached the level he has, when his skills were ready for a top career in music. He could have blown his ultimate opportunity before he was ready. The question to ask yourself is how do we apply this to your life?"

"Curt actually gave me a way of thinking about obstacles," Bob replied. "He called it "Remember and Forgive." As a surgeon, he can do everything absolutely right, but with adverse conditions still lose the patient. So he has to not only judge the outcome, but also distinguish between his performance and the outcome. He gave me this list of steps."

Bob pulled out two pieces of paper folded in his wallet. One was the process model Jeff had given him. Attached to it was an oversized Post It note that he had placed in the obstacle section of the process. He handed it to me:

1. **Do:**

Do whatever the performance requires.

2. **Analyze:**

Evaluate how you did. Look not just at the external results, but also at your internal performance. You may have done everything in your power, but still had poor results. This distinction is critical to moving on to the next performance. Did you do everything you could? If so, what could still be changed or improved? If not, how will you avoid the shortcoming next time?\

3. **Listen to Feedback:**

Listen to others, in search of things you might not have known or seen. Do not give them authority to condemn you, but to instruct you. We are after the lessons here, not the guilty.

4. **Learn and Remember:**

This is the key ingredient for future improvement. What will you do differently next time? What did you learn? How will you acquire the necessary knowledge or skill?

5. **Emotional Control:**

After you have processed the preceding steps, check in with your emotions. If you need to regroup, set some goals for yourself, so you can focus on the task at hand. You may need to postpone grieving until later, in order to refocus now. Solve the problem at hand; grieve later.

6. Process Later:

After every performance, take some time later to process exactly what happened. This goes for successful performances as well. Process in a safe environment, an environment in which you can allow yourself to be honest about what happened, and what you want "to-do-next-time-you-perform." This will also help you understand more clearly what needs improvement.

"Curt said he developed this procedure when he was a resident," Bob added. "He would be cruising along putting in sutures and the Attending Physician would not say anything, no feedback, no support. He took that to mean he was doing a good job. As he got closer to the critical sutures, he might be just as accurate, but the sutures became more and more vital to the patient's survival. They called these sutures 'widowmakers.' If they weren't exact, the patient would die. At some point he would put in a suture, and the Attending would say, 'You just killed this person.' That devastated Curt. To correct that step, he had to remove the suture and do it again. I can't even imagine the emotional pressure he must have felt trying to do that.

"He made a commitment to himself to be better, not only at putting in the sutures correctly, but also in dealing with his response when he made a mistake. He knew his response had a direct effect on his performance and his patient. He also knew that with practice he could control his response."

"What did he tell you about his fear or doubt?"

"He told me he was just like everybody else. He has times when he is afraid. He said almost everyday he doubts something. He said the important skill was to know how to deal with it. He obviously has thought a lot about it. What's great about this 'Remember and Forgive' routine is I know I can use it right away. Curt said it becomes somewhat automatic over time so it's more subconscious, but he still does it. In the 'review later' phase of it, he dictates himself a letter after every case, talking about what he did, how things went, and what he still needs to learn or do better. I've started doing that for myself. I think this will really help me with presentations."

Creating Energy

"What did he say about energy?" I asked Bob.

"That part was great. He said that the whole thing boils down to making decisions about where you get energy. Who gives you energy, and who takes it away? What activities give you energy, and which ones take it away? He has that down pat. He told me that he works over a hundred hours a week, and yet he has learned to build into his routine a way to get energy when needs it, or when he just wants to feel better about things. He spends time with his family when he can, but he makes sure that he really connects with them when he is with them. He told me how at sundown he would take his kid, Ben, down by the swimming pool and look at the butterflies and frogs. When he works out at home, he has his kids with him, and he has built them miniature gym equipment for them to play along with him. He takes them for rides in his Jeep. On weekends he bikes on Saturday and plays basketball on Sundays. He said a lot of the things you and he talk about and do together give him energy."

"I try to be one of the people who gives energy to him whenever I can. We do have a good time together. In fact, I would say a good part of my job is to protect him from educational and administrative situations that take energy away from him or the other Attendings. So how will you use that?"

"When I was driving home one day after visiting my brother, I made a mental list of the people in my life who give me energy. I made a commitment to spend more time with them, and not just have it happen by chance. My family gives me energy most of the time, but we haven't done a good enough job of making sure that happens. In the beginning, it happens by accident, but with application it can be made to happen, just like Jeff said about his performances."

"Yes," I replied, "and sometimes it comes easily. One woman at a company I consulted with told me about a trip she made to Disneyworld. She was dreading it because she thought all she would be doing would be chasing her kids around. She decided that instead of just reacting to them and letting them dictate the trip, she would view the trip as a performance. Each morning she got up and thought about how she wanted to feel that day with her kids. She knew there were a few things she wanted to do, so she kept those in mind. She didn't try to over-control her kids, she paid attention to her responses, and as a result, things went great the first day. She went back to the hotel thinking it couldn't be that easy, but the next day the same thing happened. By the third day it was even easier to do. She said it was the best trip she ever had with her family."

"That's what you were saying earlier about vacations not being escape. They have an active purpose in life," added Bob.

"Right. So your family can be a source of energy. Does that sound free?" I asked.

"Definitely. It certainly feels more like freedom than responsibility."

"What did Curt tell you about gaining energy at the hospital?"

"That was probably the biggest help. I figure if this guy can get energy in his life, I should be able to do it. He said that at the end of the day, especially after meetings that drain him, he would go look at the patient board and pick one patient to talk to. That reminds him of why he does what he does. He talks to the patients about their lives. He wants to know them as people, and learning about them gives him energy, because it reinforces his understanding of how he is helping them.

"He doesn't care if it's a farmer or a lawyer or whatever. He said that he has heard some fascinating stories. So, at the end of a day, when he's staring at three hours worth of work still left to do, he talks to a patient and re-energizes. All of a sudden, what might have taken three hours takes two hours, because he has more energy and is more focused. In the alternative, maybe he can slip home for dinner and see his family. I was impressed. I felt a little ashamed that I moan about my life. I've tried all this time management stuff, and that's important, but what Curt made me realize was that it is more about energy management. Where does it come from, how do I get it, and what takes it away? Sounds familiar."

"I know."

"I'm really starting to put the pieces together. I also understand why you started with the dream first."

"Why's that?"

"What I've learned is that it is easy to jump to obstacles and complain about things. It's easy to blame everybody else for what happens to you. Knowing what I want and what I will work for gives me something to tie the obstacles to. In a sense it gives me a direction I was missing before. I just knew things didn't feel right, but I felt powerless to do anything about it. Now I know what I want, and I feel I have a way of getting it. It is still hard. I mean I wonder if it is really possible to feel that way all the time."

"I never said you would feel that way all the time," I answered. "I had a professor at Darden Business School say something to me that made sense about all of this. His name is Jim Clawson. He teaches our process to his students and in the executive education classes. He said that you go through stages. I'll never forget a talk we did together. He opened the talk by asking a group of employees at one company what they hoped for on the way to work that morning. We got three responses. The first one said, 'I want the day to go quickly so I can get home.' The second person said, 'I just want to show up and get my paycheck.' The third response was, 'I hope I can catch up on my work and quit just putting out fires.' " Bob smiled as I continued.

"Jim grabbed me later and said he was beginning to understand a difference between himself and me, and what I'd learned about Curt, Jeff, and John. He said that the people in that meeting didn't even *believe* that gaining energy was possible. Or at the very least, they didn't believe that you could control whether those moments happened or not. He has been thinking about our process for a couple of years. He is now a several steps beyond the audience, but he hasn't quite created the environment for energy-gaining moments to happen on a regular basis. Jim said that where I was, where Curt and the rest were, was that we expect them to happen, and protect the things that create them. None of us feel the way we want to all the time. It is working for those feelings and moments, learning from them, knowing they are possible, and finally believing they will happen if you work for them. It's not just what you want, but what you will work for."

"I'm close to the believing they can happen stage," Bob said. "I feel as though I know how to learn from them, and then how to make them somewhat predictable and repeatable. I still need to tell you a story from last time that I think fits into this conversation."

"Shoot."

"OK. I decided several years ago that the family wasn't spending enough time together, so my wife and I agreed that I would build an addition onto our house. We were going to make it a family room, somewhere we could get together with the kids and their friends. So I did all the planning, took out a loan, and started building it. Now two years later, it is not even close to being finished. I just am too exhausted, and see it as work. It has alienated me more from the family than it has brought us together. I feel embarrassed about it."

I thought he was going to break up.

"It just added more pressure to my life. This thing that was supposed to feel great feels awful. I feel stupid and lazy."

"Why did you want me to know this?" He looked up at me and a small grin started across his face.

"Because I realized that it was a lot like the dream-goal thing. I figured when it was finished, we would feel a certain way. But the process of doing it has made me feel worse. What I've decided is to work on creating the feelings of family first, and that will help me want to finish it. I can involve my kids and wife in building and furnishing it. We can do it together. Curt told me that his kids think it is cool that he is remodeling the house. He went out and bought them little kid tools, and he takes them to talk to the workers. That is what I want to do. That's what I'm going to do. Maybe not exactly that, but like that"

"Great. Anything else?"

"No. I think that's it for today. I want to get home."

"Alright. Next week?"

"Sure. Hey I bought that Goo Goo Dolls album you were playing. My kids love it too. I listen to it in the car now."

"Cool."

Bob strode out of the office. He seemed to understand what we were doing. That is still a far cry from being able to do it on a regular basis. What impressed me was his ability to apply the lessons from the others and from me to his own life. He was doing the work, and that was all I could ask.

The Rhythm Of The Hills

The hills of the Ragged Mountains sloped from one to the other with such subtlety that the Specialized Road Bikes transcended the function of mere transportation. The commingling of human rhythms with the topographical cadence created a purity of action and thought that inspired us to understand and execute each nuance of cycling. Curt and I settled into what we called the rhythm of the hills. The challenge was to use the gears and muscles in harmony with the terrain. The Saturday afternoon sun eased itself into the crevice of a far off mountain pass as the pebbled country road took us under the tunnel of trees and out into the vast valley of freshly cut hay. As we accelerated around the slightly banked turns of the road, the large bails of hay watched over us approvingly like the monolithic heads of Easter Island.

Gears were shifted at a furious pace as we climbed the ridge, our bikes and bodies swaying back and forth with metronomic precision. The rhythm of our breath intensified as we completed our ascent. My hand left the custom triathlete bar to find the perfect gear for descent. As I tucked in behind Curt, the vacuum created by our closeness pulled me along. We took turns leading the way down the three-mile hill, using each other's air wake to slingshot into the front. With our backs parallel to the ground, our bodies were motionless. At sixty miles an hour, pedaling merely disrupts the rhythm, the speed. The trick is to relax, to trust the energy of the ground and the bike to do the work. This is Mother Nature's version of an E-ticket ride at Disneyworld.

A grin sneaked onto my face as we flew down the hill. Cars coming from the other direction were filled with admiring smiles. Most of them could ride the bike down this mountain, but few of them could trust the bike or themselves enough to relax and experience the rapture of a free-fall. Cars coming from our direction pass only as we slow down at the end of the hill. They flash five, sometimes six fingers at us to indicate their awe of our organic speed. Curt and I stayed low through the last bit of hill as we came into the flat valley. My muscles cramped as I fought the wind, yet attempted no movement. The slightest rise up into the wind steals speed. Sitting straight up guarantees more serious punishment, the wind strong enough to knock us to the skin-tearing asphalt.

The familiar sound of Curt's beeper interrupted the sound of our bodies whushing through the humid air. The beeper was the ultimate metaphor for the relationship between freedom and responsibility. At times, the beeper allowed Curt to get away when the hospital became oppressive. Once away, he could solve most problems over the cellular phone he kept wedged into the saddle pouch on his bike. Other times he knew he'd have to call someone and direct him to rush back to save someone's life. The beeper was electronic leash and technological emancipation in the same little black box.

We pulled into a store parking lot as the beeper sounded. While I placed the bikes up on the rack strapped to the spare tire of his Jeep,

Curt punched in the number that flashed on his beeper and hit "SEND." This time someone yanked the electronic leash hard.

"This is Curt. I was paged. Uh-huh. How long ago? Get the OR ready. I'll be there in ten minutes." He folded up the phone. He didn't say anything. He pulled off his biking cleats, slipped on his sandals, pulled on his t-shirt, and jumped up into the Jeep.

"Let's go. There's an aortic dissection waiting. You might as well come along and watch."

As we drove, Curt explained the severity of an aortic dissection. He said the probability of survival was low, but he had to try. Curt once told me that surgery was like batting in the World Series. As long as you're at the plate, something good can always happen. Curt almost always won, but when he lost, he went down swinging.

We flew through the Virginia countryside. The topless Jeep amplified the hum of the oversized tires as we turned on the interstate then down through town and into the hospital drive. We ran through the locker room and changed into the green scrubs that were standard issue. The OR sent my instincts into instant recall, reminding my body of those lonely first few months of life. Curt realized that he was still wearing his sandals.

"I'll be more comfortable," he said as we hurried into the scrub room.

I watched through the window, as the middle-aged woman's limp body was made ready for surgery. She had collapsed at her daughter's wedding. The spreading of the ribs, the blood pumping through the profusion machine made the consequences of failure clear. A person, a real live human being was lying on that table, amongst the machines and gowns and rubber gloves that moved with precision and speed.

Surgeons have been described as body mechanics. That was my first thought, as I watched them work. Music blaring, conversation about yesterday's game or tomorrow's date sometimes filled the otherwise sterile air. Little in what the surgeons do in a routine procedure reveals the life and death nature of the situation. Superficially, it might have been a '66 Mustang under the sheets, but I knew that this unfortunate woman had a daughter whose wedding day might also be the day her mother died.

I remembered a scene from the movie, "The Right Stuff." In it, a reporter suggests to test pilot Chuck Yeager that a monkey could do what these astronauts were doing. They merely sat in a capsule while NASA pushed all the buttons. Staring at the ground, thinking about the real challenge of being an astronaut, Yeager reminds the reporter that the astronaut climbs into the capsule knowing he risks death. These surgeons know that is not a '66 Mustang under that sheet. Everything that each person in that room does matters to the person lying on the table. Everything matters.

The smell of burning skin and fat blasted into my nostrils as we walked into the OR. The Cardiac Fellow was cauterizing the chest to stop the bleeding. I pulled the wire and cloth mask up over my nose to stop the fumes from sweeping further into my stomach. I was blinded as my breath fogged my glasses.

Curt seems larger in his surgeon's guise. In this arena, he had the juice, he was the man. Curt had on his game face, his eyes darting about. He walked up to the table and stood silently taking in the situation. His focus shifted from his surroundings to his plan of what was needed. Curt lets the vision of the next four hours sweep through his mind. The distance in his eyes reminds me of T. E. Lawrence as he conceived the rear assault on Akaba, across fifty miles of impenetrable desert. In my mind, I hear Curt say, "Nothing is written," as the scrub nurse pulls on his gloves.

The OR lures the most talented doctors into the demanding life of surgery by dangling the seductive attraction of emergency cases as bait. In these moments everything mattered. Each person in that room has one purpose, to do whatever is needed to save this person's life. The ultimate responsibility rests on and in the hands of the surgeon. Confronting an aortic dissection is the medical equivalent of facing a squad led by Michael Jordan or Larry Bird in the seventh game of the NBA finals. Though the odds are long, if this woman dies, the family may think it is the surgeon and his team that has failed.

As I watched for the next three hours, I thought about Curt and how different he seemed in these emergency situations. When I had first started observing surgery, I found it fairly boring. By my third visit, I thought that it looked pretty easy. I made the mistake that most people make. Surgery, according to Curt, is not about the incisions, but about making the right decisions. After being around this for eight years, I understood better. It was this simple explanation that made me understand better the idea of performance as a general concept. *Performance is the creation and expression of an idea.* Whether it is sports or music, business or surgery, the physical expression of an idea is only part of the process. Execution is important, but deciding what needs to be done is critical.

I have learned a lot from Curt over the past eight years. I think he learned from me as well. He initially invited me into his world, because he thought there were similarities between how athletes and surgeons dealt with performance. What we figured out together was that what was common was the pursuit of engagement, the rhythm of performing, and the physical expression of a mental concept.

I watched, as Curt loomed large over the table and the rest of the team. My own picture of Curt is of someone who is slightly built and in perfect condition. The first time I walked into the OR in an emergency case, however, I noticed how much bigger he seemed, how he took control, accepted full responsibility. My impression of him as slightly built was by contrast with years of playing basketball around people much taller than I. Curt was in fact over six feet tall. He looked much larger as I watched him trying to save this woman's life.

I rested against the wall. It was exciting for about ten minutes and then they settled into doing the work. I thought about Curt as my friend and how much he had meant to me the last eight years of my life. When I separated from my wife, I was scheduled to travel to Sweden. I thought about canceling, because I needed to find a place to live. Curt told me to go on the trip. He would take care of everything while I was gone. When I came back, I had a place to live, some extra money, and was invited to dinner with him and his wife, Megan, for the next six months. They turned what could've been one of the worst summers of my life into one of the best.

The Art Of Medicine

During the year following that summer, Curt and I biked over 2700 miles. We got into all kinds of things. I taught him to snowboard and rollerblade. I became his eyes and ears, reporting to him on books he didn't have time to read, or movies he couldn't see. In the summer, Curt, Megan, and I went to the beach and watched a movie every night. I chose the movies such as Lawrence of Arabia, Pump Up the Volume, Endless Summer II. In each movie, we found a take-home lesson, something we could apply to our lives.

Curt and I have grown into great friends, people who enhance each other's lives. Maybe the most important thing he has done, however, is given my work a larger sense of purpose. Curt and John Molo are responsible for getting me to look beyond sport as the only area of interest when it comes to performance. Molo suggested to me that he, too, used many things he learned as an athlete in high school when he played the drums. It was Curt who initially talked about training his medical residents and students with the broad perspective of performance. Together, we have presented seminars to some of the best surgeons in the country.

Most important of all, though, is that Curt began to see his patients as performers. His experience was that the patients who had the best recovery were also those who took control over the whole process of surgery. They took responsibility for their recovery, relied on the doctors to do their things, but actively participated in their own recovery and rehab.

When Curt and I present this, we call it, "The Art of Medicine: The Patient as Performer." Similar to Dean Ornish's conclusion that love and intimacy were the most important factors in health, Curt and I believe that balancing freedom and responsibility are of key importance for a patient's recovery. That means having a dream, a way they want life to feel after the surgery, learning and doing what they can, dealing with fear and pain, and actively recalling and projecting what they want life to be when they are better.

To allow this process to work requires a lot of time for Curt. He must spend enough time with each patient and his or her family to understand their lives, their fears, and their desires. He knows that it is a great responsibility. Ultimately, though, the freedom of doing so allows him to connect in a real way with his patients as people. He has certainly done that for me as a friend and a colleague. He has done more than any one person outside of my family to help me find the life I want.

I heard Curt talking in a hushed voice. Someone had done something different than he asked. The tension in the room was high. I remembered what I had learned on the U.S.S. Eisenhower. I had been asked to determine what made the LSO's (the flight-landing directors on board carriers) effective. It came down to two simple things: tone of voice and credibility. The pilots I talked to tell me that when they were learning to land, or when they landed under difficult circumstances, they wanted to know that the voice in their earphones was from someone whom they trusted. They wanted to hear a calm voice. The situations were difficult enough without emotions being added to the mix by some jerk on the other end of the radio. When I came home from that trip and showed Curt the photos from the flight deck, he was like a little kid, and wanted to know everything I learned. Since that time, among the people Curt and I have interviewed is a best selling author and an astronaut who helped fix the Hubble telescope. His strategy is learning from everyone he can.

The OR seemed to be back under control. My back was growing tired and I had to go to the bathroom. Part of the learning experience for residents is to learn to stand for hours, to time when they eat so they know when they will have to go, and to suppress any itches that might happen. I, on the other hand, had not undergone such training. I needed to go. I walked away expecting to hear that this woman had survived, and that the family's special day had not been completely ruined.

Later that night, I called Curt. He told me that she had died on the table. I was surprised and sad. I asked him what her chances had been going in. He told me that she had about a five percent chance of surviving. I would never have known that by how Curt or the rest of the team approached the surgery. I remembered what Curt told me about optimism and his responsibility as the leader in that room. I went to my notebook to read his words:

I believe that optimism is necessary for elite performance. I need to exude an optimism that the task before me and my team can and will turn out in our favor. In the OR, I must maintain this attitude in the face of worsening, even overwhelming odds. A quarterback must come into the huddle with the belief that anything is possible. If I don't approach the challenge in this way, my patients, my team, and I have lost before an attempt at salvaging the situation has even begun. You've got to believe, and you've got to get the people around you to believe. Without this attitude on all fronts, one's efforts in any area will most likely be lackluster, at best, and more likely, futile and disastrous. You've got to believe.

I believed in Curt because I trusted him and had seen him live his life this way. My idea is that life is, in fact, a performance. It demands that I bring that sense of belief to my own life. I'm not talking about denial of bad things, but the recognition that I can learn from the bad things, that I have some control over my life, that I will make some good decisions and recover from the bad ones. Life requires this optimism, and all the people I interviewed exhibited it, but Curt had put it into words for me.

As I got ready for bed, I thought back to a recent time when a high profile patient of Curt's had died. A young boy had been given a lung transplant from living donors. It was the first operation of its kind in the state of Virginia. Two men donated parts of their lungs to help this kid. He survived the operation, but died from complications several months later. I remembered sitting with Curt at his house in the country, listening to trains dawdle past. He talked in a whisper as he told me about the death of the boy. He took the loss personally, not because he had blundered, but because he cared.

Suddenly Curt brightened, looking right into my eyes. He told me how the boy's mother had come to the hospital a week after the boy's death. Another young boy had been admitted waiting for a lung transplant. He had no mother, and his father couldn't stay with him. The mother of the boy who died told Curt that she needed to be there for this boy, to share with him what she had learned from her son. Curt marveled at her resilience and her desire to help. Most of all, he was inspired by her desire to go on with life and to cherish her son's memory. The woman had told Curt that sitting by and mourning his loss would not be what her son would have wanted. She was making her son's life count for something by being there for the child awaiting the lung donation. "He would not have sat by and done nothing. He taught me about life. He would have wanted me here, so I want to be here," she told Curt. As I lay down to go to sleep, I pictured Curt and me sitting silently as the trains slowly ground past.

Chapter 9

Put Your Hands On The Keys

Success As An Obstacle

The following week, I was sitting on the front steps of the medical school, when I saw Bob walk towards me. He had an agenda showing on his face. That was good. It meant he was asking questions and seeking answers.

"Hey man, what was the name of the fix-it guy on The Jetsons?" he asked.

"What?"

"You know, the fix-it guy on the Jetsons?"

"Why do you need to know that?"

"I don't know. Some guys in the parking lot were playing some game, and they asked me who the fix-it guy was."

"Henry."

"Are you sure?"

"Yes, I'm sure."

"Pretty impressive. I'll bet you don't know the name of the school Elroy went to?" He thought he had me.

"Little Dipper."

"Right."

"I watched a lot of television growing up. Now that we've solved the major problem of your day, what's up?"

"Not much. I wanted to tell you that I see what you were talking about with the bad days. You know, not as many and not as bad as they used to be."

"Why do you think that's happening?"

"I feel as though I can respond better to things. I just don't let things bother me as much as I used to. I guess I also have a clearer idea of what's important to me now. I also remembered a story Hornsby told me. Sometimes I get stuck and a little tentative about taking action on something. I procrastinate because I worry about the outcome. If I look at the process," he said as he pulled out the well-traveled piece of paper, "I realize that I still tend to jump straight to obstacles, without planning out what I want and committing to do the work. Sometimes I just get nervous, like when I have to do something with the boss."

"That sounds familiar. Let me tell a story that Bruce Hornsby shared with me that really helps when I get afraid. He told me about the time he and Branford Marsalis played the National Anthem at an NBA All star game. He said he was so nervous his hands were shaking. He held his hands up above the keys, and they were just shaking. He knew Branford was nervous also. The lights were cut off and a spotlight went on them. Bruce said all he could think about was the billion people around the world watching the game on television. He forced himself to put his hands on the keys. Once he felt the keys on his fingers, everything clicked, and he was right into the music. When I find myself getting stuck I just tell myself, 'Put your hands on the keys.' I like that. It really helps. Why do you think Bruce placing his fingers on the keys was so helpful?"

"I guess he means to just get started."

"That's part of it. What else could it mean? Let's take you for example. When your boss asks you to learn something or present something, what do you do?"

"I go learn the material, and I try to anticipate any questions that might come up."

"And if you are the expert in your company on this particular project, who knows more about it than you?"

"No one."

"If it is something you really liked doing or felt you knew well, what happens?"

"Usually, I start a little slow. I look around the room to see how people are responding. If I really know the material, though, pretty soon I'm into the material and less concerned about what people think. I actually look forward to questions, because I know I have thought of most of them before they come up. I know I'll know most of the answers. If I don't, I'll know how to find them quickly."

"That feels pretty good doesn't it?"

"It feels great. It's that sense of engagement you talk about."

"Right. So by engaging the material, the activity feels better than by trying to control the nervous energy. Why do you think Bruce felt so much better when he put his hands on the keys?"

"Because they felt comfortable. He'd done the work. He could focus on letting his talent come out."

"Right. If he hadn't done the work, though, it would not have felt comfortable. In the locker room before any basketball game, players will ask the manager to bring the ball rack to them so they can hold onto the ball. It is a calming feeling to them, the leather on their fingertips. It means something. It gives them a comfortable place to put their energy. But it only happens because they have had that feeling so many times. Look, you're going to get nervous around your boss. There's not much you can do about that. But if you have a place that you feel comfortable, some source of power to go to, it eases it a bit and allows you to get into whatever you're doing."

"That makes sense. So what you're saying is that when I am doing some sort of presentation, do it in a way that I really know my stuff."

"In a sense, yes. But the opportunities are there on each slide. You want the slides not only to convey information, but to set you up to feel good about what you are presenting. When you look at the slides that way, they become a source of power for you, something like the songs Bruce plays. He knows that each song is a chance for him to show off. He knows them cold. He knows them so well, in fact, that he can play around a little bit with each one. Because he has that baseline of power, he can make himself vulnerable to the moment. He becomes more spontaneous. There's a good lesson in that. It becomes a relationship between power and vulnerability."

"My head already hurts."

"Stay with me because this is important."

"Keep it simple."

"If you have a question just ask."

"Shoot."

"Alright. When each of us is born..."

"Oh no!" Bob grimaced.

"Like I was saying, when each of us is born, we're vulnerable to everything around us. But as we grow, we learn. In fact, little kids love to learn. They are always learning, imitating, and then looking to see if they get a reaction from the people around them."

"One day my kid came to the table and started cursing. I asked him where he learned that. He said, 'from you, daddy.' Everyone laughed when you said it.' "

"Whatever. Do you want to hear this or not?"

Bob was pretty full of himself today. He just smiled.

"In imitating other people, kids gain a sense of power, of control over their environment. As they grow older, they keep imitating and learning, creating a power base from which they will operate. They keep getting rewarded, so they keep doing the things that seem the most rewarding. Pretty soon, they're adults, and they have a fairly good sense of their own power. For some people, especially people who are successful early in life, success itself becomes an obstacle. Young kids, though, have playtime built into their day. They have recess in school, or they just go play. They use their imagination. As adults we have to find time to play or we have to build play into what we do for a living. But as our responsibilities mount play drops way down on our list of priorities."

"I meant to ask you about that. Jeff has success written underneath obstacle. How can success become an obstacle?"

"Truthfully, I think success can become one of the biggest obstacles we face. Think about it. The more we are rewarded for something, the more we want to feel that way again. If the success is the only thing that makes us feel good, pretty soon we grow tired of doing it, or we reach a level that exceeds our talent. Why did you stop playing basketball after high school?"

"I wasn't good enough to play in college."

"Exactly. That was hard wasn't it?"

"It really hurt. I missed it. I played intramurals in college, but it wasn't the same. It didn't matter as much."

"But you enjoyed it right?"

"Of course. Otherwise I wouldn't have kept playing."

"Aaaahhh! So when you took away the rewards, you only did it for the sheer enjoyment of it."

"Of course, but I don't see your point."

"It was worth the enjoyment. That was enough for you to keep in shape and to face the ever-present risk of injuring yourself, wasn't it?"

"Sure."

"Look at your life now. How many things do you do for sheer enjoyment?"

"Not many."

"How about your job? Why do you continue to do that?"

"Come on! I need the money. I do enjoy parts of it though."

"And if I took away the part you don't like doing, would you do the things you enjoy for free?"

"I don't know. It depends on what other options I have."

"You probably don't even know what things in your work you would do for free, do you?"

"Not really. I don't have time to experiment. As you would say, I don't have time to have new ideas. In fact, I'm scared of having new ideas, because I don't want to lose focus on my work. I might lose my job."

"When you first started working, you thought it was pretty cool right?"

"I loved it. Being on my own. New car. I felt free."

"And now you don't love it anymore. Why do you suppose that is?"

"Tell me, Einstein."

So much for respect.

"I heard a story once about some kids who played in an old man's yard. The yard was big enough to play lots of different sports: baseball, football, soccer. Every day these kids would go over and make a racket. The old man tried to frighten them away, but they would still come back every morning and stay all day. The old man thought about calling the police, but he figured the kids would retaliate by messing up his yard or doing something to the house. So one day, the old man went outside and talked to the kids. He said, 'I'll give each of you a nickel for each day you come and play in my yard.' The kids couldn't believe they were going to be paid to play. So he reached into a jar full of change and gave each of the boys a nickel. 'Remember you have to come everyday to get the nickel,' he said.

"For a couple of weeks, the kids came to play, and each morning the old man gave them a nickel. Eventually, the kids were making less noise outside. The old man watched them through the window. One morning the biggest kid told the old man that they needed a dime for each of them to come play everyday. So the old man agreed. Each morning the kids were given a dime. He reminded them that they had to come play everyday.

"A couple more weeks passed. There was a knock at the door. The biggest kid this time said that they needed a quarter to come everyday. The old man told the boy that he simply couldn't afford that, and he begged them to keep playing in his yard. He told the kids that he would feel lonely without the sound of their voices. The older boy conferred with the other kids. He walked back up to the door. 'I'm sorry, we can't keep playing for just a dime everyday,' and he and the other kids walked away. The old man smiled as he shut the door. The kids never came back. Why do you think that was?"

"Because they started playing for the money instead of the enjoyment?"

"Right. Nothing had changed. They had lost sight of why they were there in the first place. Most people think that story is ridiculous, but variations of it happen everyday. People trade their own ideas of life, and work for money. They forget why they started doing something in the first place. For these kids the freedom of playing became a responsibility. They had to play every day. All they thought about was the change the old man was going to give them. They destroyed their own sense of play."

Power And Vulnerability

"As the rewards piled up in your life, as you were more successful, you cashed in," I continued. "Better house, family, vacations. What was once freedom suddenly became responsibility."

"We've been over that."

"But what effect has talking about it had on you? You still have fewer ideas, and you take fewer risks. You learn less outside of your job. You cling to that power base that you've been building over the years. It's frightening to look beyond it. It's even more frightening to realize that the power base can be swept away by a bad day on the Asian exchange or a bad stockholders' meeting."

"You can say that again."

"So you cling to your power. You try to build it by repeating the successes you had before. But you're not really growing. In order to add to the power base, you have to be that little kid again, looking and learning. You have to be vulnerable."

"Give me an example."

"The residents at the hospital I work with use the word "competent" to describe how they want to be and feel in their lives. At first what I thought they meant was to be just good enough or even average. That didn't seem right to me, so I kept asking them what they meant. For them, competency is not merely what they know, but having a program to learn the things they don't know and apply them effectively. When someone comes in with a problem they can handle, they deal with it. But if someone comes with a problem that is outside their power or knowledge, they have to ask for help, perhaps from someone above them in the hierarchy. In essence, they make themselves vulnerable. At your job, how do you feel when you don't know something and have to ask the boss?"

"Lousy. I don't want to ask. It makes me feel weak, incompetent."

"How about when you were in school? Did you like asking questions in front of the class?"

"No. I hated that."

"Right, so you take fewer risks, make yourself less vulnerable, and cling to the power you have. Or you go learn something on your own, and risk missing an important bit of information that someone on a project might know. At the hospital, vulnerability is built into the system. Now I'm not going to say it works flawlessly. People are still people. But the life and death nature of medicine makes the decision simpler. If the residents don't help the patient, they could die. They have to make themselves vulnerable to learn, to help the patient, to save a life. It's a subtlety of the system, but it has an important effect. The residents know they have a certain power base they can rely on. But they also know that part of their training requires them to admit when they don't know something and ask for help.

"Power-vulnerability. As a result of this system, the Attendings know that to give the patient the best care, they have to deal with questions at all hours of the day and night. Imagine calling your boss at four in the morning, because you have a problem. The Attendings know that they have to be a resource to the residents or people die. If all the Attending did was to impose power, to act like authorities, they would have to micromanage every patient, and the residents would never progress. The Attendings would never get any sleep. And people would die."

"So how do I use all that?" Bob asked. He was rubbing his head. I had to end this soon. I decided to summarize and let him go contemplate all that I had shared.

"Here's how to think about it. Success can be a major obstacle in life. You achieve things, and that builds your power base. Then you cling to that power. What was once freedom is now responsibility. The things you've acquired eat up your paycheck, and you have to be good in your job just to be responsible for those things. You worry that going away from your power base will weaken you, so you keep doing the things you can do that keep your job. No risks, low levels of learning. By focusing on your power, you narrow your vision, and you miss opportunities to grow. The trick is to hold onto your power, but to be vulnerable enough to see things outside your power base.

"The residents can't say, 'Well, I can only treat pancreatitis, so I'll deal with that even though the patient has an aneurysm.' If the patient has an aneurysm, the resident must call the Chief Resident for proper care of the patient, and to learn how to deal with the next aneurysm. The challenge for you is to figure out how to make your bosses and colleagues resources to help you to grow in a way that also benefits the company and the customers. If you don't do it, someone below you will, and you'll merely feel the breeze as they pass you by."

"I'll have to think about that some more."

"Here's one more way to think about it. If I had come to you and said, 'Hey Bob, let me teach you what I learned from a bunch of performers: athletes, musicians, surgeons, business people, actors, pilots,' you would've said I don't have time or I can't learn anything from those people. But for some reason, you were feeling vulnerable in your life. Your power base is solid, but the benefits aren't outweighing the costs. So you said something about being unhappy to your friends, they saw me speak and we end up talking to each other.

"If you hadn't been vulnerable, you would never have learned anything from a swimmer, a musician, and a surgeon, because you would have stayed focused on your power, and just kept seeking the same life based on the same successes. But something compromised that power enough to make you vulnerable. Vulnerability is our greatest gift in life. Remember, I'm talking about vulnerability in its sense of *openness*. It gives us empathy and the chance to learn about others and ourselves. The key is to hold onto the power you've already built, and stay open to other things."

"Why didn't you say that an hour ago?" He smiled.

"I'll see you in two weeks. What High School did Judy Jetson got to?"

"Orbit High." Bob laughed as he walked away.

A Dangerous Man

Working with Bob fully engaged me. I liked him, because he was not a dreamer who just fantasized about the big things in life that he would never work for. In a sense, Bob had already begun holding onto his power and being vulnerable at the same time. He wasn't taking my word for things. He allowed me into his world, and he was learning. He was educating himself. I'm not Bob, and he isn't me. We come from very different backgrounds with very different baggage. But we connected, because we had both experienced fear, a fear that our lives don't matter, that we don't count. We connected because we wanted to do something about that fear. The cost of not doing something about it was too high. It guaranteed that our lives would not count for much.

People around us would tell us how much we matter, how they couldn't imagine their lives without us. Our reality was that we had to matter to ourselves. Bob had to know that he mattered to himself.

Nothing anyone else could do could make him feel that. He had to find it out for himself. What John, Jeff, and Curt had accomplished in their lives was to be themselves, to hold onto what was important to them, and to live lives that had an impact on others. In today's society, that is hard to do. Despite all the narcissism in society, we find safety in fitting in, in being a part of something.

In a sense, we become our own benevolent oppressors. Yet these men learned to be themselves in some of the most difficult and controlling environments that exist today: medicine, organized sport, and the music industry. And they do it in a way that each of them is thought of as unselfish and giving. They create opportunities for other people. We do what we're told because it is seems safe. In the long run though, it is a pyrrhic victory. It extracts too high a cost. It costs us our dreams, ourselves.

T.E. Lawrence wrote:

All men dream, but not equally. Those who dream by night in the dusty recesses of their minds wake in the day to find it was vanity; but the dreamers of the day are dangerous men for they may act their dream with open eyes, to make it possible. [11]

Bob was becoming a dangerous man. He now knew being himself was possible. The next step was to help him come to expect it to happen, to find places that it could happen seamlessly, to create the environment that made it happen. He still had a lot ahead of him.

---

[11] T. E. Lawrence, Seven Pillars of Wisdom (USA: First Anchor Books, 1991).

Chapter 10

Learning How to Fall

Fear

I looked up from the computer and out towards the street. I could see Bob moping around, walking back and forth slowly with his head hanging. He wasn't due for another hour. I wondered what he was doing so I headed outside. I reminded myself that the last time we met he was feeling unsure of how to let go of his power base and open himself to new learning opportunities. I wasn't sure what he'd taken away from our last meeting. He seemed okay when he left, but not as excited as the other times we met. In truth, I was hoping he would struggle a little more than he had in learning the process.

It was coming too easy for him, which meant that it was still superficial, not yet acquired at a visceral level. That happens fairly often. People understand something when they sit and talk with me about the process, but they also confuse small successes with having learned something. It is another example of success as an obstacle.

Just because something worked or they achieved some result, doesn't mean they have acquired the skill or learned something truly meaningful to them. The goal for me is to help someone acquire the skill, so they can use it when the pressure is the greatest. After all, the essence of what I'm trying to share is to be able to make yourself vulnerable to the things that mean the most in life. That means greater risk, deeper potential levels of hurt, and it requires that we eliminate the excess anesthesia from our lives.

Bob had stopped pacing and was just standing there, looking at the ground. His hands were clasped behind his back. He looked like he was waiting for the bus.

"What's up?" I asked.

His head popped up. He seemed a little disoriented.

"Huh? Oh, hey. Nothing. I just got here early and wanted to think some more before I came into see you."

"Do you want me to go back inside?"

"No, that's okay. We can talk now. Can we just sit out here?"

"Sure." The sun was warm without beating down on us. We sat on the steps of the Old Medical School. Bob let out a huge sigh and then took another deep breath as he sat down.

"So what's going on?" I asked.

"I feel like I'm losing ground on this whole thing, like I'm regressing."

"Why do you say that?"

"Well, when we first started working together, I didn't really believe you, you know, that focusing on how you want to feel everyday would change your life all that much. Then when I went to see Rouse, and as I made some observations about my life, I realized that I wasn't really paying attention to the life I had. I found some freedom for myself in simple places. During that time, though, nothing was very difficult in my life. Maybe that made it easier. Recently, I don't seem to feel the same way. It isn't as exciting. Sometimes I start thinking about the people you sent me to see. I mean they lead exciting lives. My life isn't all that exciting. I start comparing myself to them, and I feel like I'm missing something."

"Why is an exciting life now so important to you?"

"I guess because of the people you sent me to see."

"I didn't send you to see them so you could compare yourself to them. I sent you to them so you could learn from them."

"I know and I have done that."

"Have you really learned the right things, though? Sounds like you focused on all the hype that surrounds what they do. What I hoped you would understand was that the fundamental aspect of what they do, of how they live, is this sense of engagement we talked about. Sure, the excitement adds something. I can tell you that many of the people I interviewed do not lead exciting lives. They lead fulfilling, engaging lives.

"I can also tell you that for someone like Jeff Rouse or Curt Tribble, the number of times they were excited is tiny compared to the number of times they might have experienced boredom or drudgery. What they talked about was creating the opportunity to engage in their lives. For most of those I interviewed, the excitement can be a huge distraction that keeps them from engaging. Those distractions can lead to poor performances, which in the long run makes everything more difficult and less fun."

"You mean like when Jeff went to the first Olympics?"

"Exactly. Most of what I spent my time doing with Jeff was trying to undo the excitement that led to pressure. I can honestly say that not one of the people I interviewed listed excitement as part of their dream. I'm not saying it can't be part of it, but the cost of excitement sometimes outweighs the good feelings it has. In fact, I don't remember you ever saying that being excited was part of your dream."

"That's true. Maybe excitement is the wrong word."

"Maybe not. Look, when you first started working with me, observing yourself, planning things, talking with your friends about these issues, it probably was exciting. That excitement, though, was probably more in the novelty of it than in the doing of it. So now we're past the excitement stage, and we can really go to work on making the engagement happen. Tell me what you've been doing."

"Okay. Well, I've been making observations and trying to list out the aspects of my dream that I've identified so far. I like the idea of engagement. I mean I feel that. So then I asked myself what does it feel like when I'm engaged. I listed those out as feeling connected, a sense of play, the presence of curiosity. Curiosity is a big part of it for me. I used to just listen to people or television or movies. Now I want to know more about why people say the things they do or how something was built. That was how I was as a kid."

"So these elements of your dream, are they all things you will work to get back into your life. Is the benefit higher than the cost?"

"I'm still trying to figure that out. So I moved to preparation. Where do these things happen for me, and around whom do they happen? That's hard to answer. The curiosity is just a part of me that I was neglecting. I didn't value it. The preparation piece of curiosity is to really listen. I heard someone say recently that hearing is physical, listening is psychological. That made sense to me, so I try to listen carefully to everything now. At work, I don't just hear what needs to be done, I listen for why it is being done. I mean, I want to understand why I'm doing things."

"Sounds familiar."

"That makes the projects more interesting and opens up all kinds of ideas for dealing with things. I also found that the more I listen to people at work, the more I understand how to work with them."

"So why the long face today?"

"I guess I have run into some obstacles."

"Such as?"

"Well, mainly myself. I have all these great new ideas, but then I start doubting myself. I start thinking, 'Who am I kidding? I can't do these things.'"

"That's understandable. Everyone goes through that. Remember the standing civil war. The desire versus the fear."

"So what do I do about that?"

"There are a couple of keys here. First you need to examine that fear, what it is that you really afraid of. If every time you want to do something important to you, don't do it just because you're afraid. If you act solely out of fear, you'll never be open and free enough to do something worthwhile. The fear serves a purpose, but the point is not to defeat the fear with the desire. The trick is to create an environment where they can coexist. The way I see fear is that it is the impetus to prepare to do all the things we can to control our environment.

"I don't think it tells you to abandon the effort. The fear protects you by challenging you, by making you go through a checklist to see if you're ready. That minimizes the fear, but doesn't eliminate it completely. Fear also gives you the energy to perform, to keep you physiologically on your toes. It triggers the 'fight or flight' response that kept us alive in primitive times.

"Reminding yourself of why you want to do something heightens the desire which then engages the fear. In developing the desire, you turn anxiety into arousal. You talked about wanting to be excited. In that case excitement or arousal is good. If it is solely caused by fear, then you feel it as anxiety-produced fear. Remember, we're not trying to win the standing civil war. We're trying to create a friendly competition in which the fear and desire push each other. The more you truly want something, the more fearful you might be about not actually attaining it. If the fear is too great, you won't even try. Then what? You've guaranteed yourself that you won't attain it."

Taking Charge

"Is there a way to minimize the fear?"

"Sure, and it's different for everybody. There is one common way to deal with it at a fundamental level. I call it learning how to fall."

"That doesn't sound so good."

"But it does help. A better way of saying it might be: if things go less well than you want, you will have a way of dealing with it for the moment.

"When I was a kid I played basketball a lot, but never really got coached. We played on the playground on hard asphalt. In pick-up hoops, you never take charges or dive after loose balls. But when I went to the high school team, taking charges or diving on the floor was expected. I was afraid of getting hurt. The coach knew that we were afraid, so he showed us how to take charges without getting hurt. He showed us the best way to dive after a loose ball.

"When you take a charge, it means allowing someone to run into you out of control, at full speed, to allow them to foul you. You have to stand completely still, or it becomes a blocking foul by you. When we were learning, we would clasp our hands over our groin for protection and then someone would slam into us on purpose. The natural reaction is to put your hands down behind you, to reduce the impact on the floor. The problem is that if you do that, you have a good chance of breaking your hand or dislocating your shoulder. The trick is to bend your knees, push away from the contact, and slide on your butt. Same thing with diving after loose balls. The idea is to land on your chest and slide towards the ball.

"Our team took a lot of charges and got most of the loose balls. I got to the point that I took pride in it. Several reporters called me crazy, but they didn't understand. By learning how to fall, I gained a huge advantage for our team, and I would do things guys on the other team wouldn't do. It looked like I was taking more risks, but I really wasn't.

"In my own life, I found ways to minimize the risk to me or to minimize the impact of falling. Again, it is all about preparation. It is the fear that stimulates the need to protect myself, but it is the desire that makes me take the risk, that gives everything I do its purpose. I really wanted to play basketball in high school. If you had said to me, 'Stand there and let someone run into you at full speed for no reason,' I would have said forget it. But playing basketball made it worthwhile. I still didn't want to get hurt, but I didn't want to quit either. The coach knew that this was a problem for us, so he shared his experience about how to fall without getting hurt. The only picture I still have from college is of Gene Banks, an All-American from Duke, when they were ranked number one in the country, with his knee at my face as I am taking a charge from him. I can look at that picture as a reminder of simple lessons in high school being played out in college."

"And all that applies to me how?" He wasn't buying this.

"In basketball some of the risk I took was physical, but the emotional risks were much harder. As I have grown older and away from competitive sports, I have applied the same principle. Let's pick something from your job, something you are in charge of. There are probably aspects of your job that you have a really good grasp of, right?"

"Sure."

"And in those cases, such as a complaint or a machine crashing, you don't worry much about it, because you know how to fix it most of the time. The people around you trust you, and you trust your people to handle some of these situations, so you don't worry about them."

"Right."

"Well, in those cases, you've already learned how to fall. You obviously have survived. I mean you still have a job, right? You've been promoted. The key is to look at how you got to this point. My guess is that you prepared well in each of those cases, and when you fell, you knew how to handle it, and each time you learned how to do it better. Not only did you know what was needed technically, but you also understood how the people around you were going to react. You processed all that, decided you could deal with the physical and psychological consequences, and stopped worrying about those things."

"That sounds right. What you're saying is that I already know how to fall?"

"Sort of. What I'm saying is that you have your own process for dealing with a fall. The tough part here is that you might be trying to do something now that seems unrelated, or you might be taking the risk alone. My guess is that your process for dealing with these things will stay the same. The stakes just seem higher because they are more personal, and they set you up to be judged by people around you."

"So what do I do?"

"The first thing is to remember the desire that you have, the dream. Then decide if you are really willing to do the work to prepare, to deal with the obstacles, and to risk the cost. You already know the process for that. Remember when I asked you to imagine yourself in the city by yourself?"

"Sure."

"You called people who you felt knew you, all of you. In other words, you had already either fallen or risked falling around these people. You probably fell, and they were there to catch you. They might have thought you were crazy for trying something, but they still loved you, still were there for you. So anytime you want to take a risk, remember who those people are. Strengthen the relationship with them to remind yourself they are there for you. The best way to strengthen that relationship is to be in frequent contact with them, and share the real you with them. Listen to them about what they want in life. Help them get it. You might even have discussions about the cost to you and to them of trying new things.

"In my case, friends are always telling me they are worried about how close I might get with someone, and set myself up to get hurt. They know I'll probably do it anyway, but they don't label what I'm doing as good or bad, unless it costs others too much. I trust their opinions so I listen, but then I choose what to do, knowing they will understand and accept me. Again, those friendships did not just happen, they were cultivated over time.

"It is not a deliberate attempt to have people there for me. It is simple friendship. But part of that friendship over time is the acceptance of each other. I take a lot of emotional risks. Having friends there makes the falls that much easier to deal with. So a good place to start is to reflect on who gives you unquestioning support. I know from our talks that you do have friends you trust. Strengthen those relationships, do things with those friends. Having them there for you is one of the benefits."

"That sounds like preparation."

"In a sense it is. I don't label making friends and developing the friendships as anything other than what it is. It doesn't really fit into a category. It is not utilitarian. Friendship is just friendship."

"Okay, what else can I do?"

"Look at all the times you succeeded in doing something that was fun or made you feel good. Look at your successes, and I'll bet you'll see that it took several attempts for something to actually succeed. This will also remind you of the role failure played in your successes. My guess is that it will be substantial. You'll see that without the failed attempts, you never would have succeeded in the long run. Learning how to fall means understanding and accepting that failure plays an important role. It might help also to go back over the times you did fall or failed, and identify the process you went through. It would amaze me if every time you failed at something, you just gave up. Look at the things you've been through successfully over a period of time, and identify the times when you failed but eventually succeeded."

"Boy, that sounds threatening."

"If we were adding up all the failures, or if we were evaluating you based on your failures then it would be pointless. What I'm trying to get you to see, is that you have fallen in the past and somehow, in your own way, you got back up and tried again. You know that set of responses, your own process, better than anyone else.

"Now here's the thorny part. Look at how many of those failures you worked harder and eventually achieved something. Then look at how many of them had the net result that you were just glad it was over. How many were cases that didn't really feel like a success. Then look at the times you failed to do something, stuck with it, and in doing so, felt pretty good throughout. Those are the ones we want to focus on. I think we'll see that in those cases your innate curiosity drove the entire activity. Instead of feeling like a failure, your curiosity took over, and you simply wanted to understand what went wrong. At its core, even failure creates opportunities for your curiosity to engage you."

"Hey, that's right. Like when we couldn't fix a car when I was a teenager. We didn't get down on ourselves. We just kept trying to solve the problem. To solve it we had to look deeper. I guess you're right. I do have a means for dealing with falling somewhere in me."

"The final piece of this is that you have to keep looking inside yourself. Turn your curiosity on yourself. Why do you care about some things and not about others? What are you really afraid of? If that gets too uncomfortable, I'll send you to someone who deals with that."

"Sounds good. I have to get going. Thanks a lot. This really helped."

"Sure. Remind yourself that you have to ask yourself the right questions. You can call me when you have to, but if you get down again, solve the problem. Remember why you want to do something. Weigh the benefit-cost. Talk to your friends. You just started applying this process. Be patient."

"Alright."

Bob strode down the stairs and up the street. He still moved slowly, but together we had re-engaged his curiosity.

Chapter 11

For The Children

Facing Fear

I met Bob after work one day at the same bar as last time. Lisa and Mark were with him again. I walked in, said, "Hello," and ordered the usual draught Bass.

"I've been thinking a lot about the things we talked about. It makes sense to me, but doing it is awfully hard," said Lisa.

"That's true. I'll repeat the question "What will you work for?""

"It made me wonder, though, if trying to feel a certain way all the time is all there is? I mean it sounds kind of selfish to me," Lisa said in a questioning manner. She had really thought about this. There was no sense of attack in her voice. She honestly wanted to know more.

"Let's think this through. When you're angry, feeling unfulfilled, disconnected, how do other people experience you?"

"What do you mean?"

"If I ran into you one day, and you were angry, what would our interaction feel like to me? How do you think you would affect me?"

"Probably negatively. I don't think you'd want to be around me."

"Right. So how you feel affects other people. Now how about your performance at work. How productive would you be if you were angry?"

"In the short run, I can use that anger to be productive and sometimes that feels good when I'm finished."

"Does that give you a sustainable energy?"

"No, I'm just glad I'm done. I'm usually exhausted."

"And how do you feel the next day?"

"I usually feel drained. It takes a day to recover."

"So in the short run anger can work. What if I said to you that from now on I want you to get angry everyday, so you can be productive everyday? Would you do it?"

"No way. I'd go crazy."

"Exactly. How about being afraid, feelings of fear? How do they affect you?"

"The same way. I am more timid though. Actually, a day doesn't go by that I don't feel afraid of something."

"What do you do about it?"

"I try to ignore it. When I can't, I just wait for it to go away. I'll go for a run, or talk it over with a friend."

"Then the next day starts and the fear comes back."

"Sure."

"So you ignore it and you build some things into your life that protect you. Yet you never deal with what's causing you the fear."

"Well, I feel helpless against them, as though I can't change them. I'm too locked into my life the way it is."

"And the way it was. A lot of our fears come from past experiences that we haven't learned from. I'm not a therapist, but I 've seen enough frightened people to know that what they are afraid of today is likely to be based on something they've experienced in the past. I'm not talking about huge traumas. I send those people to experts. I'm talking about feelings we've had of inadequacy, of disappointment. We don't want to feel that way again.

"When Michael Jordan got cut from his high school team, he said to himself, "I never want to feel that way again." And what did he do. He improved on what was right about himself. He did the work. It was worth the risk to him because he knows what basketball feels like when he is engaged in it. We all get afraid. The question is what do we do with that fear?"

"What do we do with it?" asked Mark. He was not saying much. I think this was hitting home with him. I wondered if it made Bob see the Vice President in a different light, more human, more like himself.

"I can only tell you what I've learned and what my experiences have been. What you do is up to you. This is a difficult part of the process, because I have to be careful not to open people up too much. Dealing with the fear is as important as nurturing desire. My experience with it is that unless we deal with the things we are afraid of, they show up throughout our lives. They accumulate and then one event or experience can bring out the cumulative effect. I'm not sure if we ever really get rid of the fear completely either.

"What I've learned is that being afraid tells us we need to improve, we have some work to do. Too often, people focus on the single incident that brought the fear to life. The work they do is to minimize the impact at the moment, but they don't really improve. They maintain status quo. Then they try to avoid those situations in the future. The problem with that is that sometimes the greatest fears surface around the things we also care about the most: relationships, safety, our jobs."

"That sounds familiar," said Lisa.

"So what *do* we do?" asked Mark a little more perturbed this time.

"What I've learned is to face the fear head on. I had to ask what makes me afraid? Some of those things I couldn't eliminate in my life. What I could change is how I experienced them. I'm not talking about positive thinking. It goes back to doing the work. Benefit-cost. If I'm really afraid of something, and I know that eliminating it from my life costs too much, I have to come to grips with it. I learn from the experience. If I have a fear of failing, what can I do to minimize the risk that I will fail? I usually can't change the people around me, so I have to do something about myself. I have to improve my skills, my ideas, my execution of whatever it is I am doing.

"That goes for any kind of fear: snowboarding down a mogul run, riding my bike at 55 miles on hour down Afton mountain, being in a relationship, or giving a presentation. There is a certain skill set I must have to make it happen the way I want it to. But knowing the skills is not enough. You have to have the skills developed enough so they become automatic. You have to do the work. All that brings us back to making observations, finding your passion. Some people don't have what they want in life, and they complain about it. I listen and ask them why they think they don't have those things. Usually they blame someone or something else. One of the people I interviewed was Fred Haywood. He was a national swimming champ, he set a world speed record on a sailboard, and he now sells real estate in Hawaii where he grew up. He told me a story that I think about sometimes when I'm tired of doing the work, of putting in the hours.

"Each day he would go down to the docks to watch the fishermen come in and show their catch. One of the ships that came in fairly often was something to see. It was beautiful. It was shiny and always spotless. It had all the high tech gear on it. Every once in a while it would come in with a good-sized catch. The captain and the crew would always make a grand entrance into their slip. All hands would come running to see the ship's catch. It was exciting and showy. There were times, however, when the ship did not have any fish. They had caught nothing. There was no show, no excitement, no success.

"One night he hung around the docks late and saw an old beat-up ship come home quite late. He could see the captain picking his way through the dark. The crew looked content as they went about their work. When they unloaded their catch, Fred couldn't believe how many fish they had on board. It was great. It too was exciting, but it was exciting for a different reason.

"He asked the captain about it, and he told Fred he was aware of the other boats coming in earlier and showing off for the tourists. The captain said, 'I am a fisherman. I like to catch fish. It's what I do. Always keep your hook in the water. If it is in the water, you will have a chance to catch something. Keep it available. Give yourself a chance to be successful.' "

"Fred said he never forgot that lesson. Whenever he could, Fred went back to the docks after dark to watch the captain bring in his catch. He almost never came home without a good catch.

"I've often wondered why people like Fred, like Curt, Molo, Jeff and all the other people I interviewed who had similar obstacles, didn't give up. The answer seems simple to

me now. They had found their passion, just like the fisherman. It wasn't about celebrity or showing off a shiny boat. It was about doing something they loved. They had tried other things, other ideas, but they knew how they felt when they did certain things. If they didn't feel that way after a legitimate effort to learn something, they focused their energy on something different."

"They kept trying until they found what they could love, not only when they achieved something, but also when they were in the midst of doing it, or of learning about it. One question Curt asks people when they are deciding on a career is, 'What do you love learning about?' If you don't love the learning part of something, then you will probably not be engaged by it as competition increases. Once they found things they loved doing *and* learning about, they became engaged.

"That is what allows these people to put in incredible hours. They also realize that they need to hold onto the reason they do something, whether they hit an obstacle or achieve success. If they hit an obstacle, they have to re-energize themselves. They have to remind themselves that the benefit outweighs the potential cost. It is an active process. If successful, they then remind themselves of what their motivation is, so that celebrity or the success itself does not seduce them. If they forget why they do it in the first place, if they stop learning, if they aren't engaged in the activity itself, they might substitute the success for the activity itself. And success is external; it is a fickle mistress."

"How does that relate to the fear?"

"The distinction between external success and internally energizing activity ties back to fear, because success cannot do much to contain fear, and the engaging activity can. When they feel afraid, they can actively go back to what reminds them why they are doing what they're doing, and draw strength from it. That is a subtle difference. If you merely focus on the fear, you do something to avoid it, to make it go away. You stay one step ahead of it. But if you remember why you're doing something, and it is meaningful to you, if it comes from inside you, it gives you a reason to confront the fear. You are not avoiding failure. You are reaching higher, striving to live the way you want. Avoiding fear never fulfills

people. That's too superficial. Knowing why you do something, and what you want out of life is energizing. It gives you a reason to do the work that is sustainable. It produces sustainable energy."

"Give me an example," said Lisa.

Picking Them Off, One At A time

"I've just started working with a good friend of mine, Benita Gras-Thompson, a nurse. I'll use her as an example, because she has experienced something new recently that led her to talk to me. She was a runner in college and burned out. She got tired of the rigors of competition. She loved running, but the organized competitions, the coaches, and the pressures drained her, so she just quit.

"About six months ago, Curt got her to go biking with him one day. She loved it, and with her running and swimming skills, she decided to start entering competitive triathlons. It turns out she was quite good at it. But five months later a lot of the same pressures that she felt in college running were building up. She had won a several races, and had decided to try out for the Chilean National Team, her home country.

"Suddenly she had to deal with coaches again, and her focus drifted to winning, or even not losing. It began to lose the quality of play it had had for her. That drained her, and made her life much more difficult. So we started talking. My first job was to remind her of why she had started competing again. She had made the National Team, and she had beaten the best Chilean women, so she had earned a chance compete in the South American games, representing Chile.

"She placed fourth in South America. From no time to big time in six months. It could have been overwhelming. As a nurse, she works twelve-hour shifts, but she still has to train every day. She gets up at four in the morning, runs and swims, goes to work for twelve hours, and then bikes on her trainer at home for an hour. That would kill just about anybody. As the trip to Ecuador for the South American Games closed in, things started to get to her. She also had to work more days to make up for the days she would be gone. She was physically exhausting herself and emotionally challenging the play aspect."

"Whenever I talked to her, I'd let her vent for a while to blow steam. And then I would ask her one simple question: 'Why are you going to Ecuador?' She would close her eyes and a big smile would break out across her face. I'd ask, 'What are you thinking about?' She would say she was picturing herself down on her handlebars and focusing on the person in front of her. She was picturing picking the leaders off one by one. She loves that feeling. That feeling is powerful enough for her to put up with all the preparation and all the obstacles. Just like Rouse talking about Easy Speed, that feeling was something she could experience just by visualizing it.

"At work, Curt helped her by teaching how to gain energy from her patients. When she left for Chile she was nervous about competing at a high level. So she would picture talking to some of her patients, and how they inspired her, especially the heart and lung transplant patients. In many hospitals, doctors and nurses serve as a reminder to the patients that they are sick, but getting better. Curt and Benita go in with a different mind set. They are going to help the patient to reclaim who they were before they were sick, and to help become what they want to be when they return home. In doing that, they helped change the patients' outlook, and brightened up their mood. That in turn inspires Curt and Benita."

"Wow," said Lisa.

"My brother Dave did mention those two, and how much fun it was to talk with them," said Bob.

"How's he doing?" I asked.

"Great. You would never have guessed he had bypass surgery a month ago."

"Benita has made the decision to learn more about competing at a higher level. Her goals are to shoot for the Olympics, and to be one of the best in the world. But her dream is that feeling of competing, playing, getting down on her bars, and picking off people one by one. Without that feeling, without the play, she will never make it. It is just too hard. As she does the work and grows more fatigued, the fears taunt her, just like the rest of us. She worries about losing, about not being good enough. She worries about those times when she has to tell people she didn't win.

"If all I do with her is keep pumping her up, she will become dependent on me. If she doesn't face the fears and deal with them, acknowledge that they might never go away, she will never reach the level she wants to reach. She wants to compete at the highest level for two reasons. One is the experience of being really good, and all that brings with it: the travel, being part of a national team. But she also wants to compete at a higher level, because the challenge keeps her growing and learning, and that forces her to focus more on the feeling of playing to win. She has decided that her dream is important enough to try and face her fears, and she is doing that work. I have sent her to talk with other people who deal with that. But at this point, the risk is worth it to her."

I'm Not An Athlete!

Mark jumped in. "Well, I'm not a surgeon or nurse or triathlete. "How does that help me?"

"Your task would be to find comparable moments in your own work, in your life, and to structure your days around them whenever possible. I'll give you another example, but it's a long one. Want to hear it?"

Mark nodded.

"The process I have been describing works not only for individual performers, including business people, but also for organizations of all kinds.

"Near the end of my father's twenty-seven year career as an executive in the Federal civil service, he was faced with a major challenge. In 1992, under a Senate mandate, his Department established a new unit of twenty people, reporting directly to the Secretary. The unit was to coordinate all activities aimed at reducing the occurrence of lead-based paint hazards for children in the nation's older housing. As the only available senior manager with relevant experience, he was designated unit director.

"The Senate saw the Department as either dilatory or inept, or both, in its previous lead-paint activities. To some extent the Subcommittee's views were justified. HUD had made progress, but there were undercurrents of resistance. There was a very costly 'remove-all-lead' program being pressed by children's advocacy groups. Those in the Department with the mission of affordable housing for low-income families saw the removal proposal as a huge cost obstacle to their own mission.

"The Senate's directive was viewed by the Department's management as punitive, for it gave it no additional dollars or staff for the new organization. Implicit was the direction: take the resources out of your research office, which the Senate believed was resistant to the lead mission. The research office reacted defensively. It transferred twenty people, out of a staff of 140, those it deemed least needed. They were seen as "the culls." The transfer selections were made without consultation or choice for those affected. Those not selected for transfer were seen as "winners;" they had made the cut. Those selected had a right to be upset by the way they were chosen, and the implied slur it cast.

"The new unit was off to the worst possible start. It was an unwanted appendage in the Secretary's office. It was a costly threat to the principal mission of the Department. It was a castoff and potential rival to the office of research. It had to prove itself to a hostile and suspicious Senate and to public advocacy groups. And it was seen as a terrible 'why me?' mistake by its new staff.

"As the director, my Dad saw dismal morale as the paramount problem. If left untreated, it would make all other efforts fruitless. He was initially viewed by his new staff as the enemy 'them,' part of an unfeeling management that had done them in. Fortunately, he had been friendly with most of them for many years. The tide began to turn when they learned that he, too, had been designated for transfer without consultation. He became one of "us," when he successfully bargained for the return to the research office of three persons with especially difficult transfer problems, and then recruited three "winners" voluntarily to replace them.

"It took many kinds of actions to turn around the morale problem, but establishing a "vision" or "dream" for the Office was the most effective. Lead-based paint technology is a dry and abstract subject. Detecting its presence in wall paint requires sophisticated radiation instruments that measure the radiation reflected back from the lead in the wall paint.

"Abating the hazards requires a very long timetable of planning and repair work. Setting goals and missions based on the detection and abatement of hazards would not be enough. Those goals would be too slow and too impersonal. What he needed was something more immediate that would have greater meaning for the staff, a vision and purpose they could work towards with enthusiasm.

"Within a few weeks of the formation of the unit, my father rented a bus and took the entire staff, secretaries and all, to Baltimore for a day visit to the Kennedy-Kreegar Clinic for Childhood Lead Poisoning. He wanted everyone to see, first hand, the effect lead has on children, to see the palsy and the neural impairments, to see the bewilderment of children too young to understand why they hurt. That trip made clear that *the unit's fundamental mission was to help children avoid such risks.* Detection and abatement were just intermediate steps towards the protection of children. By taking his staff to the Clinic, he exposed them to ideas that compel action. The dream was about helping the kids. With that vision in place, the unit jelled.

"For example, once its general training had been seen to, the staff took another course to prepare for licensing by Maryland, a leader in the field, as lead-paint abatement professionals. Again, all twenty, including secretaries, participated. Fourteen passed. At the opportunity for a re-exam, the six who did not receive their license vowed to study more diligently, and to pass 'for the honor of the unit.' All did.

"There were other things. He personally designed and paid for 1000 colorful lapel buttons for the staff to wear and to pass out. It had the familiar circle with the diagonal slash through it, over the letters Pb. Pb is the chemical symbol for lead, so it was shorthand for "no lead." It was a handy identifier for staff, and a good message to pass to the people they worked with. But time and again the staff came back to the dream, help the children, when they had to make choices among alternative courses.

"Over time, the staff performed wonderfully. Congress no longer saw the Department as dilatory. The advocates worked with them, not against them. The mission offices of the Department accepted the Lead Office as prudently balancing affordable housing with lead abatement.

"The question for you," I said to Mark, "especially as a leader, is what opportunities exist for you to create that staff dream. Who are your customers? Who are the final consumers of your product? I have to believe that in the mortgage business there are plenty of people whose dreams you help bring to life."

"So you're saying the process is something you can also use for groups?" asked Mark.

"Sure, but if you only focus on the group, then you will be unlikely to succeed. The group dream is only as strong as the individual dreams that make up the group. I was surprised at this result. When I first started working with people, I, too, thought it was only for individuals. But as I was asked to work with teams and with groups, I realized that two things were being accomplished at once. Two needs were being satisfied. The first was the individuals' need for independence, the need to have their own identity through the development of their personal dreams. But second, and just as important, was the individual need for connection, to feel a part of something good.

"Instead of fitting in, people could find the right fit. They had responsibilities to the group, but they were free to fulfill their responsibilities in ways that fit them. That combination of factors is what I think is meant by team chemistry. If the group's dream acknowledges the individual's dream, then the individuals will work hard for the group. When it becomes the 'do it my way or take the highway strategy,' people get defensive and start focusing on anything they can do to keep some piece of themselves, like the staff my dad was assigned. But he found a way to bring a personal meaning to the work. The staff saw him as a resource, who helped them feel good about what they did, and to become engaged in their work. He wasn't just an authority to whom they reported, waiting for marching orders.

"This sounds obvious and useful now. I have had similar experiences at work with people. The truth is it never originally occurred to me how important the individual's dreams might be to the group. I was always taught that we had to have a work ethic. The company was a resource to people merely by paying them.

"And yet every study out there shows two things about money relative to work. The first is that a salary that is perceived to be inadequate by an employee is a great source of dissatisfaction. But the second is that money is not the principal positive motivator or source of happiness for people. So by paying people enough money, you might keep them from being unhappy or dissatisfied, but that alone doesn't create the enthusiasm needed for an organization to compete at higher levels. Again, a subtle shift, money can be a demotivator but not a prime motivator. That subtlety has an enormous impact on the type of company you have. If I asked you to describe the qualities of a great team, what would you say?"

Lisa and Mark thought a minute. "They work together, they are enthusiastic, they help each other. If one person falls behind, the other people pitch in to help. Competition exists, but it is more with other teams, than within the team. Actually, there is healthy interaction within the group. I guess you would say that people are playing to win, to be better, but not to beat the others by tearing them down. They have a clear sense of purpose, and of what they are trying to accomplish."

"I would agree with those characteristics. What strikes me about that is that most of those are internal qualities, or at least internally and emotionally driven. So can you see how a person feels at any given moment might have an effect on others, on the group?"

"Yes. I get it," said Lisa.

"Let's go back to fear. If people are constantly afraid of losing their jobs, of not fitting in, of letting others down, how will that affect the team?"

"Not very well. I know when I feel those things, I tend to withdraw and limit what I do to exactly what I'm told. I think I'll make fewer mistakes if I just do that," sighed Lisa. Mark was deep in thought again.

"Sometimes you will have to do what you're told," I said, "but you can prepare yourself to be ready for those moments when you can break free. John Molo is a professional drummer. He has played for Hornsby for 20 years. But he also likes doing other gigs. He will go to a local bar to play with a Latin Band, even if there are only five people in the audience. He told me that when he first started playing with Bruce, he learned as much as he could about the music Bruce listened to and played. It was an incredible amount of work, but John knew that when Bruce wanted to take the music in different directions, he would be ready. He not only knew the music but integrated it into his own tastes."

"Bruce and John would tell you that they have both been lucky, but they made their own luck by being ready for the opportunities that might come their way. Howie Long, the football All Pro, told me once that he never wanted to look back, and be haunted by something he didn't prepare for. These performers all found ways to make the work fun. They found the meaning in what they were trying to accomplish, and they experienced that meaning when they were preparing or dealing with obstacles. I'm not saying you shouldn't do what you're told. In fact, do what you're told, but don't settle for that. It is not enough. Learn why you are doing it. What is the end result? What is the meaning to you and to the people around you?

"For you three as managers, the challenge is to build that inquiry into your every day life, so it happens almost without effort. At the same time, build that environment at work for the people around you, the people for whom you are responsible, the people on whom you ultimately must rely. In order to do that, you need to know what's important to them. And that is difficult, because not many people themselves know what they want. It takes time and focus. But my experience is that it is worth the effort. It feels great, it has a bigger purpose, and leads to results beyond what you might have thought possible."

"How have you used this with groups?" Mark was learning now.

"I've done some consulting with companies and had success with it, sure. I'd rather give you a few examples from my interviews, though. An old teammate of mine from college had run into someone we knew in college. My teammate said that this guy was now the President of Earthlink, the internet company, so I called him up and asked him to tell me his story. It is a great example of what I'm trying to tell you.

"Several years earlier, he had a roommate who was a CEO of a company. He was frustrated one night and sat down with my college friend and they talked about how they thought work should be more fulfilling, not simply a place that supported other sources of fulfillment. So they decided to list the characteristics of a new company, a company whose function was to provide fulfillment to employees and customers. They listed things like work should be fun, not boring and stiff. They emphasized the experience of their employees and their customers.

"Well, this CEO quit his job and decided to create a company around them. He did not even have a product or market or anything else. That was the beginning of Mindspring which was eventually purchased by Earthlink. My buddy was named President. He eventually stepped down in the company because he had triplets and wanted to spend more time with his family. Check out their website and you'll see this list of characteristics still prominently featured."

"Wow!" said Andy and Bob. Mark was impressed but tried not to show it.

"Another guy I interviewed was the International Chairman of Goldman Sachs. His name was Gene Fife. Great guy! In fact, I interviewed him because I heard his assistant tell someone that he was the kind of boss everyone should have. I had no idea what he did or who he was, but I wanted to talk to him. When he first got out of college, he joined the Air Force and worked in close proximity to Neil Armstrong, the astronaut, and Chuck Yeager, the famous test pilot. Gene told me that watching how they went about doing their work was fascinating. He decided he wanted to be as engaged as they were. He did not believe that would happen in the Air Force, so he went to business school, then worked for Goldman Sachs.

"He went to New York and then was soon asked to move to California to create a presence for Goldman Sachs. He was successful enough that years later he was asked to go to Europe and improve things there. The year he went to Europe, Goldman lost one hundred million dollars. When he left, the European offices were contributing forty percent of Goldman's overall profitability."

They all stood silent. I was enjoying this.

"So I asked Gene how he accomplished this. He basically told me that leadership mattered, that listening mattered, that helping people get engaged in their work mattered. He was turned on by launching the careers of the people who worked for him. He loved that. It energized him. How did he do that? By understanding what excited the people he worked with and then helping them head in that direction. How they felt about what they were doing day to day mattered. It directly impacted the bottom line.

"I suspect he learned that by watching Neil Armstrong and Chuck Yeager. He saw their energy, their love for what they did. He internalized that and put it to work for himself, instead of merely imitating it. Then he passed that onto the people he worked with. Most of all, he loved doing the work. Not everyday and all the time, but enough to gain energy from it. I think most people feel work takes energy away from them."

"You've got a lot of stories," Mark quipped. He did not want to give in, but he was really listening. I could tell by the look in his eyes that he wanted to know more, but was still holding back. He was leaning in trying to hear every word. I knew he would go home and think about his life as a leader, as a manager of people.

"Yeah, well, I committed to learning from as many of the best people as I could."

"So give me an example of how you've used it in your work," asked Lisa. She really wanted to know how to do this.

"The best example I can give you comes from the work Curt and I have done at the hospital. Several years ago Curt was asked to run the education of the medical students as they came through a twelve-week rotation on surgery. He hired me to help him with that and the administration of the residency. We started with a very simple philosophy: that learning is more important than teaching. The medical students have a responsibility to the school and to their patients. Those could be well defined and monitored.

"The question was how to inspire them to learn what they needed to learn, while working long hours in surgery, and holding onto their reason for being a doctor. Only about five percent of the students go on to be surgeons. For many of them the lifestyle of a surgeon is undesirable at best. While they are very motivated to be good doctors and good students, the lifestyle they would endure for twelve weeks was a huge obstacle. Add that to the reputation surgeons have as being arrogant and demanding and you have students dreading the rotation."

"We put the process in as the main way of doing things. In order to do that, we had to know why the students were there, why they wanted to be doctors. Gene Fife echoed this about his work at Goldman. Why were people there? We needed to know what they were willing to do, to work for, and we needed to identify the obstacles to their dreams, and to the fulfillment of their responsibilities.

"Every twelve weeks a new set of students arrives. We ask each of them to stand up publicly and tell us why they want to be doctors. The stories they tell are amazing and touching. Most of them want to connect with people in a meaningful way, and they are willing work long hours to do that. In medical schools, a lot of things are done simply because they have always been done that way. Once we knew their dreams, and the work they needed to do, we sought to eliminate obstacles that served no real purpose. I asked the students to tell me all the things that got in their way. They came up with twelve that really made sense. I went to the Chairman of the department and asked which obstacles we could get rid of. He said that nine of them could be eliminated. I went back to the students and explained that we could eliminate those and why the other three were necessary. Surprised and gratified, they accepted that.

"In the years we've been doing it, performance has become significantly higher by any quantitative measure. We win more teaching awards, and the students are more engaged in an experience that is inherently very difficult. We hold to that standard, by learning as much as we can from the students in each rotation. Most of the changes we have made have come from their suggestions. At its core, we have given the students more freedom, and they have more willingly accepted the learning responsibilities that come with the duties and privileges of patient care.

"Curt is the face of this. He meets with the students, inspires them in a graceful manner. He goes to great lengths to tell the students how important it is to take care of themselves, to engage in their work and their patients. He knows that how our students feel, how your doctors feel, matters. As a result, he is often asked to be their Baccalaureate speaker. I work more at the policy and problem solving level. How do we structure the course so we increase the likelihood the students will be engaged? That's my job. We've moved away from lectures to doing hands on procedures such as learning to tie knots. Then I debrief these experiences with the students. I am sort of a firewall. I deal with the students who are not so engaged, who are struggling. From class to class, the students might not even be aware of the changes or of the commitment to an environment that nurtures their dreams of patient care. It is not important for people to know what I do because it is not about credit, but about accomplishing what we set out to, creating a learning environment and a culture of performance."

There was a long, uncomfortable pause. I was losing them. I had rambled on too long. It was time to go.

"Well, I have some thinking to do. Plus if I want to feel the way I want to I have to get home to the family. Thanks, Doug." Mark seemed genuinely grateful.

"No problem. Just call me if you have any other questions."

"Thanks. I will."

We split up in the parking lot. Bob thanked me again. Lisa seemed as though she wanted to talk more, but just said "Good night."

Love

I left the bar feeling pretty good. Bob's coworkers seemed like nice people. I was happy that they had thought about our previous discussion. I loved telling them the story about my father and his work. I felt a sense of pride in him and from what he had taught me. As I drove home, I thought about my parents and my sister. Sometimes I feel guilty that I can't purge my feelings concerning my adoption, but I have accepted that the feelings I have are a part of me.

It is interesting that my fears, my feelings of not being lovable, are so powerful. I wish the love my real family has shown me, and that I have for them, were my default feelings, but I have accepted that, at least for now, they are not. Intellectually, it makes sense to me. My guess is that animals and humans are programmed first and foremost for survival. We have a built-in mechanism, fear, that signals danger. The power of the 'fight or flight' syndrome is very strong. It has played an incalculable role in the survival of our species.

I want to believe, I have to believe, that somewhere inside us, is an equally powerful capability for love. I recently read Dean Ornish's book

Love and Survival.[12] He made me think about my own life. Ornish wrote that from his own studies, and those of others, he had come to the conclusion that, "...love and intimacy are the most powerful factors in health and illness." He added that he was, "...not aware of any other factor in medicine, not diet, not smoking, not exercise, not stress, not genetics, not drugs, not surgery, that has a greater impact on our quality of life, incidence of illness, and premature death from all causes." That is an incredibly powerful statement, and it made me wonder about by my own relationships: my failures as a husband, the fact that I am again single at thirty-eight, and the effect my feelings of being unlovable have on my own health.

If our instinct for fear is more evolved or more socialized than our instinct and ability to love, we need to question ourselves and carefully examine our lives, in order to thrive. Thriving and loving take work. That was what I learned from my interviews. Loving someone, loving what you do, loving yourself, can take work to hold onto. Maybe that is what is meant by a labor of love. Maybe it is just a question of our early experiences, and not merely instinct. I can't answer that. My experience is that I want to love, I want to be in love, but actually showing those emotions was difficult for me for a long time, because of the power of my fear.

The moon skirted the edge of Buck Mountain as darkness set in. My geese friends, who flew over my house every night about this time, appeared in the distance, the familiar honking capturing my attention. Even geese stay together. My mind returned to the most important and successful relationship in my life, my family. The truth is that my Mom and Dad are my best friends. I thought about the struggles we'd been through and realized yet again that the only problems we had ever really had were my doing. They went back to the adoption.

When I got divorced, I hunkered down, while at the same time beginning seriously to look at my fears. I wasn't aware that I was withdrawing. Maybe what I was actually doing was working on myself first, without letting my family know about it. If so, it wasn't deliberate. I still was a survivor, a reactor, and with those came the behaviors of withdrawal. It was simply habit. I was facing my fears, learning to accept parts of me and how they affected the whole of me. Around most people, I showed the changes, and became less the warrior and more the poet. I argued less, listened more, and got great satisfaction out of helping others, without the expectation of anything in return.

---

[12] Dean Ornish

My family, though, knew me very differently. I wasn't aware of this, however. I assumed that they saw my fear, my feelings of inadequacy. My extended family is a smorgasbord of divorce, death, remarriage, and adoption. I knew they saw me as untouchable, distant, the athlete, as much of the world did. I assumed at some level that my dad understood my pain, because his father had also left him when he was very young. We never talked about it, though. I assumed my sister understood my feelings, because she, too, was adopted from different parents. We never really discussed our feelings.

Larisa

I pulled into the driveway, sat back in the Jeep, and cranked the stereo. Van Morrison lamented his life, the song, "Why must I always explain?" drifted on the wind, echoing off the trees that surrounded my house. Man, I knew what he was talking about. Sometimes coming to this house was hard. It reminded me of the only woman I have ever truly been in love with, Larisa. We had lived together for a year while she finished grad school. From the beginning we had discussed marriage, but I knew it wasn't real. Delaware her home, was calling her, pulling her. I was a temporary interruption, but the cry was too powerful. I have trouble getting her out of my heart because she is the only person I feel I have had real intimate physical and emotional sharing in the act of love. I had always struggled with sex as one more human activity that wasn't safe for me. Wasn't I the product of irresponsible sex, my internal struggles the ultimate result?

I don't remember when Larisa and I first met, but I remember when I fell in love with her. We stayed up all night at a conference one night and talked about our fears. Her life growing up was more difficult than mine, but we shared similar feelings. We both got in our own way trying to get what we wanted out of life. As the night went on, I realized that something was changing in me as I talked to her. I could feel her making my walls fall away. She introduced my mind to my heart, my soul to my intellect. They merged, and I didn't have to hide behind my intellect or feel wary showing her my fears. When morning came, I knew I was in love.

As I sat in the Jeep, the cat she had left behind jumped into my lap. Raige was huge compared to my other cat, Boo, but he was not very tough, and avoided fighting at all costs. Boo, on the other hand, looked for fights and terrorized Raige. They seemed to have reached an understanding to occupy different parts of the house. I knew Raige missed Larisa and wondered why she wasn't here anymore. As I stroked him, I thought about how much fun Larisa and I had together when we vulnerable to each other, and not caught up in the distractions that daily life dished out.

She was a successful field hockey player in college, and we shared a love of playing and competing. Together we discovered the motorcycle game I had taken Bob to play. Most of all, Larisa showed me what I really wanted in life, the synthesis of my feelings, my body, and my intellect. Maybe this is what I mean by rhythm or engagement. Her presence might have enhanced that for me, but knowing that is what I want has helped me create it for myself. All of me, in the moment, doing the things I love and dealing with the things I don't.

Larisa allowed me to share with my family what I really needed from them, and what I wanted to share with them. I had to show it to my Mom and Dad first. I wanted them to see me as I saw myself. I remember sitting in a restaurant with them and fighting over something stupid. My dad pissed me off. He commented that I had not passed through the developmental stage of seeing beyond myself. I thought he was saying I was selfish, although later he explained that it merely limited my view and kept me from really finding my fit in the world. I got up and walked out of the restaurant. My Mom chased me down the street. It would have been funny, if I weren't so mad. She told me she loved me, and we needed to work things out, and asked me to come back in. We paid the bill (well, my dad paid the bill) and we drove home.

I opened up to them and cried. I told them about my fears of being unlovable, of feeling inadequate, of waking up for thirty years wanting to kill myself, of the horrible nightmares. I could see in their faces that they understood. Their minds were thinking back to my temper tantrums as a kid, to the times in school when I threw up, to the sheer will I applied to sports. They felt responsible for not knowing, for sending me to a school away from my friends as a kid, for setting me up for emotionally difficult situations, in the name of what was socially expected. I tried not to blame them, but I didn't know any better growing up. They were my world. Until this moment, I had no idea how to help them understand. I knew that they wanted to understand, and that was enough to start the conversation.

My mom told me more about myself as a baby. She said that when they adopted my sister, she fit right into the family. If my mom picked her up, she just molded into my mother's arms and chest. When they got me, though, I was different. She told me I never cried, and that when she picked me up, I would go stiff as a board. She remembered telling someone that I was such a good baby, and that I never cried. I could see her eyes well up, when she told me that the friend said I didn't cry, because I was scared to death. She told me about the time when I was starting to take baths, and how she tried to towel me off. I fought with her, demanding to dry myself. She gave in, and then I complained that she was supposed to dry me off. I was in a standing civil war even as a child.

My mom doesn't like crying, because it leaves her unable to continue talking, so she quickly shifted to funnier stories of how I would sleepwalk in the middle of the night. Once when we lived in a split-level house, they were having a dinner party when all of a sudden drops of water came falling to the table and floor. They looked up and saw me dead asleep, leaning against the railing, slowly peeing over the edge. She reminded me of how I used to wake up in the morning with a wet bed, but mysteriously dry pajamas. One night she stayed up and watched me as I climbed out of bed without opening my eyes, unaware of where I was. She laughed as she saw me drop my pajama bottoms, pee in the bed, and then crawl back in. Embarrassed, I smiled, feeling like a four year old again.

My Dad mostly listened. I knew he heard what I was saying. He was thinking of solutions and eventually researched psychiatrists who dealt with the special issues I faced.

My father was a latchkey kid who grew up in Manhattan. His love was stickball. He had shared stories of growing up in a city, swimming under the George Washington Bridge, and having someone steal his clothes. It forced him to pretend he was a world-class distance runner, passing through the city streets, hoping his underwear looked something like track gear. He served in the Navy aboard the Missouri right after World War II. He went to Harvard on the GI bill, and then continued on at the Harvard Business School. He loved to learn and valued his intellectual ability.

On the other hand, my parents knew I hated school, and never pushed me, because they knew it would merely drive me further away. But my dad and I, as far back as I can remember, shared that love of learning. It was how we connected. Whenever I bring friends home, they are amazed at how we can sit at the dinner table, talking long into the night. So many people have said they wished they could have that with their dad. I knew it was special.

I needed him to hear about the other side of me: my heart, my fear, my pain. Not surprisingly, he wanted to know everything. I remember wondering why I hadn't done this earlier, and what I had missed for so many years by assuming they knew all. They had always loved me and reached out, but I had never been able to tell them what was in me. At times growing up I blamed them for not knowing. Our lives together were always based on love. They were always there for me, but there was always a distance in me.

Larisa, without knowing it, had shown me what I wanted, what I'd work for. She showed me not just a piece of me, but how all the pieces fit together. I think it was that illumination that made me believe she was the one for me. Without her, though, I could still share that with myself and with the people I cared about. Since that point, my life makes more sense to those around me. They understand when I don't want to participate in societal rituals, when I want to talk, or when I just need to be alone. They really know me, but only because I know myself and share that knowledge.

When I talk to people about what I had with Larisa, I describe it as a sense of "us." I am disappointed in how many people who have been married for years, tell me they don't know what that feels like. How could I continue to feel sorry for myself, having something so many people haven't even experienced? My feelings for Larisa have not changed at all. Letting go of what we had is still hard. But it is not as hard as knowing that I wasn't strong enough to do the work that all relationships require, or to even try. I'm not saying relationships of any kind should be work or feel like work, but doing the work is a fundamental part.

When I talk to my mom about her marriage of more than fifty years to my father, the smile in her voice conveys the satisfaction of the complete engagement of two lives sharing everything. The true power of their relationship shows through when she talks about the work, the tough times. The smile in her voice doesn't falter, is not diminished, when she describes the difficulties they've been through so many years together. She understands that the work is also an expression of love. In fact, maybe that is the purest sign of love, when it is truly connected to something larger; two lives entangled and intertwined, messy but real, culminating in a transcendent "us."

Larisa wouldn't do the work for me. My insecurity wouldn't allow me to do it alone. I don't think she knew how to include others in the work. She needed to do the work with her family, but still she was trying to do it alone, instead of inviting her family into the process.

Larisa helped me include my family, but she couldn't do the work for her to include me or to include other people in her own life. As we tried to remain friends, it was difficult for me to let go of what we had.

The belief that I wasn't good enough to work for "us" transformed an expression of our deepest soul into a passing meteoric moment or just another teardrop in the rain. Larisa found comfort in novelty and newness, in her relationships. She didn't want to work through problems. I know from others that she wants friendships to be easy, simple.

Like everything else in life, relationships can be very simple. We make them hard by holding onto past beliefs and habits. We are our own greatest obstacle. I don't hold any for blame her. I have absolved her from the accommodations we couldn't make, and I think she has absolved me, but we haven't forgotten. We learned the lessons, but she couldn't apply them to our friendship, and I couldn't if she couldn't. What I know with certainty is that we can't have what we won't work for.

As we tried to hold onto some connection, things grew more difficult. Maybe I couldn't see her as anyone other than what she had been to me. The term "friends" never began to capture what I experienced when we were together. Over time, she found what she needed at home. She stopped returning calls or responding to E-mails. Our relationship turned into an effort. I think she forgot who I was, what made me different from other people. The technological advances of cheaper long-distance phone calls and E-mail couldn't capture the intimacy of personal communication.

We seemed to draw inferences of a calculated coldness, as a result of the intervening machinery that twisted concern and deeply felt pain into a kind of attack. The touch of our hands, the stroke of her hair, the hug that pulls us back together, were lost over fiber optics. Worst of all, those contacts with her were felt viscerally, "in my stomach." The warm feeling of "living in my chest" with her became as distant as the many miles between us.

My candid expressions of frustration were seen as weapons meant to hurt her, to challenge her. I became just another former boyfriend showing hurt and anger. In the end, she denied that "us" had ever happened. She had mistaken the light I brought to her, for that inner place she really loved. I had merely illuminated where her love belonged, not with me, but in the strong woman inside her, and with the little girl she had hidden so long ago. My role in her life was reduced to observer, or even threat.

In trying to live my own philosophy, I struggled to learn from this. Someone once asked me in a workshop how can I be so forgiving of people who have hurt me, how can I forgive myself when I make a mistake? I gave a simple answer, one consistent with Curt's idea of Remember and Forgive. I think we all have a responsibility to learn the lesson in every failure, in every hurt we cause someone else, or that someone causes us.

I know somehow I had hurt Larisa, but she never told me straight out how that happened, or what I had done. I can only guess that when I needed my own distance, when I was losing myself, she thought I was threatening to take what I had shown her away. She was afraid that without me, she wouldn't have herself. As our relationship deteriorated, she stood fast, holding onto the pieces of her that she could remember. I became a threat to what she had fought so hard for. Too caught up in my own needs, a need for that sense of "us," I lost sight of what she needed.

The lesson for me is that "us" is about two whole people, not merely each part-person providing what is lacking in the other, and certainly not about a fear of loss. Throughout the relationship, we empowered each other too much, not by giving the other what was needed, but through fear, a fear arising from mutual ignorance of each other's inner longing I never learned how much I meant to her, that she worried about losing me. She never understood the cost to me of knowing she would someday have to leave, of knowing I would have to let her go. She couldn't empathize with the fear, the knowledge I had that the end was always edging nearer.

When she finally did break away, the hole left by my absence ultimately was smaller than she feared. I don't think she'll forgive me, because she doesn't know what I've learned. She read my words then and now with disdain and with hurt. Too often, I wrote from my stomach, showing the fear and the hurt, yet free of any intention other than to help her understand what her departure cost me. Ultimately, everything we shared, any belief she had in my philosophy, in me, was lost because we both stopped living what we preached, at least in dealing with one another. In the end, perhaps even from the beginning, the trust that we would be there for each other simply dried up, leaving only the ashes of a fire that once warmed us.

Sometimes the greater powers that be send you a signal that things must come to an end. To prolong things might destroy the entire experience, pictures of times past might elicit humiliation and distrust twenty years hence. A week after Larisa left, she called me early on a Sunday morning. Her Grandmother had died in the middle of the night. I asked her if she wanted me to come up there to be with her.

She said no, she didn't need me, that hearing my voice, knowing I was there for her was enough.

A few days later I told my mom and Claudia, another good friend, about what had happened. Both of them said "You should have jumped in your car and gone." I argued that she said she didn't need me. I explained that her mother didn't like me, and that I was the last person her mother would want under foot. But when I talked to Larisa again, she complained I wasn't there for her, that she had wanted me to drive there when she called. It was just that she didn't want to have to ask.

What did my mom and Claudia know that I didn't? How could I have been such an unperceptive male? How could I have been anything else? Maybe under different circumstances I would have gone right away. Once again, I gave into the feelings of fear, of not wanting to risk being somewhere I wasn't wanted, not wanted by Larisa, by her mother, or her family. I was confused, because I had offered, and I felt I had complied with what she said, even though I wanted more than anything to be there for her. I just didn't think I was wanted.

I drove up and attended the funeral. It was hard to sit in the hotel alone, to show up at the services, embarrassed by my role as onlooker, as someone from the recently abandoned past, certainly not of the present or future. I don't think Larisa ever understood what that cost me, or what I hoped to gain. I lay in bed in the hotel racked by nightmares of not being good enough, of feeling a failure, of once again not getting it right. The demons of my childhood danced around my mind. The visions taunted me, mocked me. What makes you think they want you here? I went to the church, and I cried as I sat alone, unable to comfort her as she wept. I cried for myself, as well, feeling unloved and unwanted.

When the funeral procession drove through town, my car was the last in the line. It seemed appropriate. I would be there for her, even if I were the last person she or her mother wanted to see. At least she had the choice. Driving my convertible with the top down, I had taken off my suit jacket so I didn't sweat. We pulled into the cemetery and I paused while other people parked. Then God's signal of the time to move on came splashing down. It hit the nice white collar high up on my neck. I looked in the mirror to realize that some bird had left his latest meal, fully processed, on my nicest shirt. No matter how hard I tried I couldn't diminish the bright brown spot. It was too high on my collar for my coat to cover it.

So for the rest of this somber day I walked around with bird crap on my collar. I should have sensed that this was the end, the last chance I had to show Larisa I cared. I mustered all my courage and participated in the burial, and later at the celebration of her grandmother's life, conscious at all times of this Scarlet Letter on my neck. If people didn't know I was the former boyfriend, the desperate guy trying to hang on, surely this made it clear to all. No matter how well we dress something up, no matter how fondly I might have remembered the past, a little crap can bring clarity and focus. I should have paid attention.

The lesson I learned was that intimacy without trust cannot survive. I was reminded once again that the light I might add to the muted brilliance of someone's soul is only a part of me. It is a light that is attractive, but blinding as well. I was left wondering how to be trustful when someone tells me they love me, but when I know they have not seen all of me. The light of what I do and how I live, may be too bright. But it may illuminate only the desirable side of my standing civil war. The fear skulks in an unlit corner, seeking cover.

I thought I had learned this lesson as a basketball player, when people had responded to a physical prowess, ignoring my emotional needs and fears. I was reminded that love that hurts is also the only love worth fighting for, because the hurt and the joy are the only protection against complacency and boredom. And, oh yes, I learned that when I get dressed in my best clothes, I should keep the top up on the car.

I thought about all the people I interviewed, about the work they had done to hold onto themselves through their difficult times. All of them had something special about them, tempered by doubt. They all talked about having people around them who knew the good and difficult sides of them. They knew they weren't perfect and shared that understanding with a chosen few. Those people served as mirrors when things were tough or felt out of sync.

They had an idea of what they wanted, they prepared themselves and the people around them to go hell bent after it, and they knew where to go when things got tough. Their friends and family served as reminders of what was real, and what was possible. My family had always wanted to do this for me even when I didn't let them. What I was learning was to allow them into my life, to share everything. My relationship with Larisa was the most memorable step in this progression, but it was the interviews and the self-examination that created the opportunity.

Several of the people I interviewed told me that they made their own luck, which they described as preparation meeting opportunity. I truly believe that is what happened with Larisa. Several years earlier, I would have missed the chance to be lucky. Maybe I could have made the connection with my family without her. Maybe my soul would have eventually met my intellect without her. The truth is I owe her a great deal for making these introductions possible and timely. She helped me by being herself, by sharing what was right within her. That is why I love her so much. That is why my mom and dad will never forget and will always love her, too. I hope someday she learns to love herself in the same way. I wish I had been more complete in loving her, in showing her my feelings, but I wasn't ready. Showing that love wasn't automatic yet. I still had more work to do, to actually put into practice what I knew. I forgot to pay attention to me, to her, to "us."

The stars were ablaze in the country away from the city lights. I laid my head back and looked straight up. Someday I would learn more about the stars. Maybe not. Maybe knowing about them would take the romance away, disrupt the mystery. Knowledge can destroy that sense of wonder some times. Maybe that is what happens when people see beyond my light, my desire, when my behaviors give in to my fears.

Family Reunion

The bright moon over the lake reminded me of the beach. Nearly every year, my family headed to Southern Shores in North Carolina. That was my beach. We have been going there for thirty years, and seen it grow from run down little shacks to multi-million dollar homes and stores. Several years earlier, Larisa had joined us for a two-week vacation. My aunt and uncle and cousin were also with us. In the past, I would have felt they were an intrusion on time with my family. I came to accept that they were part of my mom's family. Their presence made her feel more complete. My father had no remaining relatives. His mother was the only one he'd known, and she died before I came onto the scene.

This particular year would be different, though. I wanted my mom's family there. I wanted to talk with them, to learn about myself from them, to share the real me with them. Larisa and I sat with my sister, Chris. Larisa knew I was uncomfortable, and she rested her legs across mine on the couch. She held my hand as I talked. She knew it was important to me that she be there. She also knew she wasn't really part of the conversation, so she let us talk. I told my sister everything. Two moments have really stayed with me. The first was when Chris told me she was afraid of me, and that my cousins were also. I couldn't believe that, but I had heard that from others, who said I intimidated them. I never saw myself that way, but I could see that when I felt threatened, I pushed people away with my physical presence and my intellect. I could argue people into submission.

This acknowledgement by Chris led me to tell her how I saw myself. I knew I had abilities, but I never thought I could fit in or be good enough. Everyone seemed to expect so much of me, expectations I never lived up to, nor really wanted to live up to. Chris, on the other hand, didn't stand out when we were growing up. She went through life being Newburg's sister, which really hurt. I told her that I considered her one of the most successful people I knew. She thrived as a wife and mother. She was raising three great girls. She had the things that were missing from my life. Most of all, she never felt unloved or unlovable. I knew she doubted herself at times, but her relationships with her husband and my mom reminded her of what she had, and what she was capable of. Compared to me, she was living her dream. She started to cry and gave me a hug.

Since those experiences, I have made a conscious effort to be honest with people about myself. I probably tell them more than they want to know. They trust me and are rarely surprised by the choices I make or the actions I take. This single bit of preparation has improved my life more than anything. The small acts of intimacy and vulnerability supported my dreams and the work I was willing to do. I have great friends. What was a good relationship with my family is now incredible. People often ask me where I call home. My response is wherever my parents are.

I shut off the radio and headed inside. I missed Larisa. Breaking up was really hard for me. I felt a deep sense of loss and of self-doubt. I knew in my heart she had needed to leave Charlottesville and return to her home ground. In some ways, she needed to share with her family, what she had helped me to share with mine. She needed to be home to do that. I wish I could have helped her the way she helped me, but I wasn't the one to do that.

After a few months away from each other, of not talking, she E-mailed and told me she missed me. She realized that what we had was great, but she still didn't have herself. She needed to find that before she could share it with anyone else. Mostly, though, she admitted that she left because of her fear, not because of me.

We never got back that sense of "us," and our attempts at friendship turned bitter. I hope she has forgiven me for not letting go easily, for standing my ground, for not being able to be friends. She told me that my gift to her, the light that shined in the dark corner in which she hid, outweighed the hurt. I wish I could say that was enough. In the end, though, she walked away distrusting, fearful of me.

Claudia once asked me what I would have wished for. That's a hard question to answer. I know in the long run, we weren't meant for each other. The trust we needed of each other, the belief we needed in ourselves, just wasn't there. Our sense of "us" was only strong when we touched, when we had a firm grasp of each other. We were afraid to find out what would happen when we let go, unable to try again once our connection was undone. What I want, what I hope she knows, is that I will be there for her no matter what she needs, no matter what the cost. She once made me promise that I would never leave her, because everyone important to her had left her as a child, if not physically, then emotionally. I know she'll never come looking. I hope, I try to believe that in her heart, she knows that all she has to do is ask, and I'll be there. Ultimately, that is what friendship means to me.

I played with the dogs for a while and headed upstairs to read. I was thankful for the time with Larisa. I was grateful for what I had learned from all those around me: my friends, my family, and the incredibly helpful people who had allowed me to learn from them.

I was applying what they had shown me in my own way, on my own terms. I was the final judge of whether or not I was getting the life I wanted. My life definitely had a rhythm to it. It carried the knowledge of how to learn, how to look at myself in an emotional mirror and see what others see. I was learning from the past. I could forgive myself and others. I was enjoying the moments of engagement, and I was improving from the failures. Best of all, I was preparing for a fulfilling future, ready to grab the opportunities I might have let slip by, but for the people around me, but for the work I was doing for myself.

Chapter 12

The Good Husband

Something's Missing

Bob called me late one night and wondered if we could meet the next day. He said he was struggling with something we had not talked about yet. He said he couldn't say what it was. I agreed to meet him for lunch. We decided to meet for sushi.

Times had really changed in Charlottesville. When I first came here twenty years ago, the big meal was a one-eyed bacon cheeseburger. I had never heard of such a thing, but my Kentuckian teammates, Jeff Lamp, Lee Raker, and Terry Gates, swore by them. They also taught me that Mountain Dew was the beverage of choice for washing them down. Now I was eating raw fish.

Bob and I sat down at the sushi bar and watched the guy slicing and dicing the fish and rice. It was pretty amazing the preparation the chefs went through to make something served raw. His name was Shige, and he was fun to watch. He flipped the knife through the air so easily. Bob moved his chair back a bit just in case.

"Thanks for meeting with me on such short notice. I just felt unprepared to deal with something that happened yesterday. I also knew I couldn't let it sit."

"No problem. What happened?"

"My wife just seems so unhappy lately. Yesterday she came home from work and had no energy. She seemed depressed. That's happened more often lately. When I asked her what was wrong, she couldn't really pinpoint it. She just felt sad, like something was missing. I asked her if she meant something was missing between us, and she said it wasn't about us, it was about her. I felt kind of selfish asking her about us. Then I got sad too, and I just shut down. I knew that wasn't the right thing to do, but I couldn't stop myself. Then she was worried about me."

"Why do you think you shut down?"

"Like I said, I felt selfish for asking her about us. It came across as though I wasn't concerned about her, that I was only worried how it affected me. Maybe that is what I meant. I don't really know."

"Sorry, Bob, but I have to be up front, by saying that I'm certainly no expert on relationships. I'm single right now and divorced. So anything I tell you will be what I've learned about from people who seem to be in good relationships over a long period of time, like my parents. I feel as though, intellectually, I know how to talk about relationships, but finding or creating the right relationship has eluded me to this point."

"That's okay. I guess I'm learning that you don't have answers to hand to me. I just figured we might talk it through, and I could come up with some ideas on my own. We haven't talked much about my marriage yet, so I wouldn't expect you to know everything about it. I guess I'm just like most men. I just don't know what women want."

"I'm certainly not going to claim that I understand women. I'll tell you this, though. I think I understand men even less."

"What do you mean by that?"

"I've had a lot of conversations lately with friends about relationships, and more specifically about marriage. I'm amazed at how few people I know who are in good relationships. One interesting aside, though, is that most of the people I interviewed were in strong, long-lasting relationships. I don't think that is an accident. So I went back and looked at some of the things they told me. What I realized is that they live the process twenty-four hours a day in all their relationships, as well as in their careers. I should have realized that early on. It just wasn't a focus of mine."

"You didn't answer my question. Why do you think you understand women more than men?"

"Oh. Sorry. Well, I can only tell you what I see in the people I work with. First of all, I have worked with far more women than men. They just seem more inherently interested or connected. It takes longer to show men that the touchy-feely aspect of what I do is important. Again, anything I say is based on my experience with people, not on the research that's available. I think about these things to apply to my own life. So keep in mind, I'm single."

"Okay, okay. Just answer the question."

"Women seem to understand better the value of friendship, of dreams, of feelings. They seem to hold onto those things longer in life. The sad part is that they tuck those dreams away, but don't necessarily give up on them in their heart. It goes back to what I said about the dream-goal distinction. The way many women were raised is not based on goals, but on community and of feeling connected. Society has set up lots of ways for them to feel connected, without having to achieve some goal. Keep in mind this is changing. The last class at the medical school was 50% women, and I can see things starting to change. The women athletes I work with are more goal oriented than the other women I've talked to."

"So why do so many feel that men hold them back? It sounds like they do what you're trying to teach me."

"Think benefit-cost. The cost of holding onto these feelings of connection is that they sacrifice themselves for their kids, their husbands, and their friends. The feeling of connection many of them get is from helping other people. Women seem to me to be far more willing to help someone through something without setting a deadline or goal. They focus on that feeling of connection, but the price is really high, when we get down to their individual dreams."

"I feel like I am doing that. I mean I sacrifice a lot for my family and the people at work."

"But you do it for different reasons, and you get something different out of it. You feel responsible and that's it. That is why it's dragging you down. You measure success by how well you reach your goals. Remember when we first started talking, you told me that you thought if you played by the rules, if you achieved your goals, then life would feel great?"

"I remember."

"I think that many men feel that way when they are growing up, Many of them think their goals are possible, and when they reach enough of them, they expect life will be great. The reason many men reach a mid-life crisis is that they do not fulfill the expectation that reaching their goals will result in life feeling a certain way, whether or not they deal with the emotional cost along the way. So men have a limited optimism, for a number of years, that the next achievement will be the one that makes their life better. They connect with others by the cost of their toys, even if they never have time to play with them. For most of the men I have worked with, this hasn't seemed to work."

"Sounds like you understand me pretty well."

"It's not that I don't understand what they do. I don't understand why they do it. My guess is that setting and achieving goals gives them a sense of purpose. But all you need to do in any company is realize that you are part of a hierarchy that has a limited number of upper management spots. It doesn't take a genius to figure out that most of the people you compete with are only going so far.

"I'll also bet you that there are technical people in your company who don't want to be promoted. They want to keep doing what they enjoy. They just want a raise every few years, and recognition of their value. They probably are like that, because they can engage in what they do, or they have reached a comfort level that fits their lifestyles. When I sold software I knew several people who turned down promotions to be managers because they wanted to keep selling. They liked it."

"There are people like that at my job."

"Curt Tribble and I have talked a lot about this. Have you heard of the Peter Principle?"

"Yeah, but I can't remember exactly what it is."

"Basically it means being promoted to your level of incompetence. Curt and I have decided that for a great number of people who experience this, it is unlikely that they were incompetent or not smart enough. They just didn't like being shifted to management functions. Men don't feel free to turn down such promotions, because they see each advancement as the thing that might change their life. That reluctance or ambivalence about managerial promotions is occurring more often now than it used to, and good companies are working on ways to compensate employees in a different manner. If I had to guess, I would venture to say that the mid-life crisis that men go through coincides with some of these unwanted changes. That is when they begin to realize there is no rainbow, no pot of gold, or that gold isn't fulfilling enough."

Women Know

"So how are women different?"

"I think things are changing, but many women I've talked with experience a similar crisis earlier in life. They just don't make a crisis out of it. They sacrifice their individuality earlier and more consciously than men. I think they know there is no fatted calf, or at least that it isn't as fulfilling as men expect it to be. I think many of them understand that.

They were not the ones taught to believe reaching external goals or material things will make life wonderful. Although for a long period, the goal of getting married for women did carry some of that weight, not as a loving relationship, but as a way station in life.

"The result is that women currently seem to have fewer externally imposed goals, and the goals are more attached to their dreams. They just don't feel as driven to do something about it. Again, that is changing as career opportunities broaden, but we still haven't come to grips with the role of mothers in society. Many are still torn by the conflict between being a mother and working. Men feel guilty about not being there enough, but society accepts that more easily."

"So men and women are different how?"

"Lets' keep it simple. Men think that by achieving a series of goals they will reach a finish line, or at least a slow-down line. They are taught early in life that they can make things happen, if they just work hard and play by the rules. Women aren't as distracted by such goals, because many of the same opportunities just aren't there for them yet. They are also mindful that at some point, they will want to raise children. So by having less freedom, they are actually less distracted by the things men pursue.

"I'm not saying it is easier or better. I am sure women would rather have the opportunities, the ability to make their own choices, and the confidence that they can achieve them, than to have limited opportunities. It think our society is in a major transition phase where both men and women are learning to deal with and exercise freedoms that weren't available to our parents."

"So what's all that got to do with relationships?"

"Society still expects most women to get married and have kids. Society still teaches men that the way to be responsible, is to take care of your family through the accumulation of things. If men don't do that, they are considered weak. If women don't marry, people ask them when they are getting married, or when they will have kids, if they are married. What's missing in all of that?"

"I'm not sure. I guess it would be what the individual needs or wants."

"Right. So people marry and chase their goals, raise their families, and continue to accumulate, so they can pass something onto their kids.

You're 45 and you're seeing me, because you don't know what you want out of life, right?"

"Yeah, but I have a better idea, now."

"Sure, but it might change, the harder you look. What we're trying to do for you is to identify your own method of getting what you want in life. To do this you've had to challenge your beliefs and your actions over the past 20 years."

"That's right."

"So what effect do you think that will have on your kids and your marriage."

"I hadn't thought about that. I figured it would be a positive one, but now that you ask, it could be pretty damaging. I mean I tell my kids get good grades, work hard. I guess I've been telling them that, because that is what I was told."

"Well, you're certainly not going to tell them not to work hard or not worry about grades. The question is why do you want them to get grades and work hard?"

"Knowing what I know now, I'd say so that they know what's out there, what's possible, and not be foreclosed from any of it by poor performance."

"Right. So that they will have choices. If they understand that the choices are not just about money, but about engagement in a dream, coupled with reasonable financial responsibility, they will probably be better off 30 years from now. So how would you apply all this to your marriage?"

"Wow, that's more frightening to think about. I start feeling selfish again. I guess that what I really need to do is to ask my wife what she wants her life to feel like."

"Remember, I can't tell you what's right. You need to figure that out for yourself. The way to do that is to try things out, and see if they are useful to you. I am more concerned about finding useful ways to think and to act, than about being right. Why did you say earlier that you didn't understand women?"

"Probably because they seem so mysterious to me."

"My point is that you don't need to understand women, plural. In marriage, you need to understand *your* wife. Maybe you can worry about understanding other women later, but the most important woman in your life is your wife. Did you ever worry about understanding your mother?"

"No."

"Why do you think that is?'

"I never thought of her as a woman. She was just my mom."

"Why do you think you saw her that way?"

"Because she was my mom. She took care of me. She was always there for me."

"Exactly. She understood you, and for you that was enough. Do you think her life was more than just being your mom."

"Sure, but I didn't spend a lot of time thinking about it."

"She probably got a lot out of taking care of you. I used to be the same way with my mother. When my grandmother and grandfather needed care, she was always there to help them. My father and I watched her go to great lengths to care for them. She always said she wanted to do it, and I believe that, but it drained her. My dad and I still don't understand it, but we have stopped trying to get her to ease back on such burdens. For her, they are not burdens. It was then that I understood my mom, and how much she could have aged raising me, and worrying about me. I never thought that it might not be the whole of her. She was just my mom. It is great to see her and my dad enjoying their retirement, and balancing with the rest of the family the care of my grandmother."

"Why are you telling me this?"

"If you just saw your mom as your mom, how do you see your wife?"

"Oh. I see your point. Now I feel worse."

"Maybe you should. I don't think so, though. Even though she works a full time job, you still feel it is her responsibility to keep the house and take care of you."

"I guess."

"She probably accepts some of it and gains energy from that. But it is also probably not all of her. What has she sacrificed to fulfill that role? What is missing from her life?"

"She said she doesn't know."

"Then offer to help her find out. Let her know that you're there. Listen to her. Ask how you can help. Here's the snag though."

"I knew there was one coming."

"One of the best ways to help her is to be whole yourself. Keep working on you. Part of working on you is playing a role in her life, not just as a husband, but also as a friend. One important thing I've learned, is that I can't let actions a friend takes have the same impact on me that similar actions my parents took. I'm pretty messy. If someone tells me I'm messy, or asks me to pick up something, I get anxious. It is not about the friend, it just stirs up how much I hated being told by my parents that I had to clean up before I could go play hoops. The friend's comment has nothing to do with that.

"I make a conscious effort to remember why I am in a relationship with someone. The hardest part for me is the adoption stuff. A woman can trigger the feelings fairly easily. When I was married, I couldn't make that distinction. It was all about my wife, not about my past. As I learned more about myself, I could deal with the initial pain, and not blame the other person. So if your wife has a similar role in your life that your mother had, there may be some triggers you need to deal with. If you'd like, I'll give you the name of a counselor to help you work some of those things out."

"What did the people you interviewed tell you? Remember you're single so I can't rely on what you do."

"Good point. If I had to summarize, it's that they weren't trying to fill a hole in themselves by getting married or being in a relationship. The other person actually makes their life better by being a separate whole person. In some cases, they became whole together, but didn't hold each other responsible for the missing pieces. They worked on themselves and shared that understanding with their partner."

"I really want my wife to feel the way she wants to. I mean I wouldn't wish what I felt on anybody. I guess I did just see her as my wife, just like I saw my mom. Funny, I certainly married my wife, because I thought of her as a woman. She really has made my life better. It got tougher, though, as we worked harder and had kids. That makes me feel ashamed."

"So do something about it. You said you had a new engagement ring. Did you give to her yet?"

"Sure did. She loved it, but that initial excitement didn't last long for either of us."

"So you re-engaged, but your view of her is still as a mother and a wife, not as a woman or another person?"

"Exactly."

"So how do you want to see her?"

"As the woman I married, the woman I fell in love with."

"Do you have many opportunities in your life to experience that?"

"No, mostly we are always doing family things."

"What kind of gifts do you give her?"

He turned red. He was embarrassed. "Mostly things to make her life easier. Practical things."

"For years and years my Dad has given my Mother fairly expensive jewelry. It never made sense to me. It didn't seem like my mom to me. But she loved it. She and I actually argued about it once. I just didn't understand. Gold and diamonds seemed like a waste of money. I thought my mom was more practical than that. Now I understand. It makes her feel like a woman. It shows her that my Dad still sees her that way. Maybe that's why they have been happily married for 47 years. Every once in a while, the old man gets it right."

"So why didn't you learn that from them?"

"Ouch! Good point. I can't say for sure, but my best guess is that until I resolved my adoption stuff I was getting into relationships for the wrong reasons. I was trying to fill a hole. That put an incredible burden on the other person, and they didn't even know it. How could they? I didn't know it. Usually, they weren't in much better shape, either. I was filling a hole for them as well. We seemed to be self-selecting. It wasn't really love. There wasn't much to protect. My marriage lasted 9 years, but it was more from hanging in there, than being in love, or feeling connected to another person. Let's get back to you. I have to go soon. Has this been helpful at all?"

"It's given me a lot to think about. I think the main idea is to keep learning about myself and sharing that with my wife. I also need to let her know I'm there to help her figure out what she wants."

"If she wants your help. You might just need to give her space and to listen to her."

"I guess what you're saying is don't try to teach her this stuff?"

"Right. What we're doing is about you, helping you identify your own process. When it becomes yours, it's Process with a capital 'P.' If you're changing for the better, my guess is she'll ask you why that's happening. Then share it with her, but don't try to get her to do it. We'll cross that bridge when we come to it."

"The other thing I'm really going to work on is treating her like a woman, the woman she wants to be. I actually think that will rekindle something in me."

"It has to be her idea of a woman, not just yours. Try some things like flowers. or little surprises, or just sitting and talking. Make observations. You'll see it when she feels that way."

"Thanks, Doc."

Chapter 13

What Will You Work for?

Our deepest fear is not that we are inadequate. Our deepest fear is that we are powerful beyond measure. It is our light, not our darkness, that most frightens us. We ask ourselves, who am I to be brilliant, gorgeous, talented and fabulous? Actually, who are you not to be? You are a child of God. Your playing small doesn't serve the world. There's nothing enlightened about shrinking so that other people won't feel insecure around you. We were born to make manifest the glory of God that is within us. It is not just in some of us; it's in everyone. And as we let our own light shine, we unconsciously give other people permission to do the same. As we are liberated from our own fear, our presence automatically liberates others.

- Nelson Mandela
  1994 Inaugural speech

The Bathtub

My time with Bob was winding down. I needed to find out where he was, what he had learned. So I invited him out to my house again to wrap things up. We climbed to the top of Buck Mountain and looked out at the Blue Ridge. We'd carried some water and Balance bars with us. It was final exam time for both of us. Had he learned what I had tried to offer to him? One danger is that I'm never quite sure if the person has heard or learned what I was trying to teach. That is why my emphasis is always on learning and rarely on teaching. the process is about discovering what's in **your** heart, what's right about **you**, and then using **your** mind, spirit, and body to work to experience it. I told this to Bob and then shared a cautionary tale about learning.

"When I was first married right out of college, my wife and I had two huge dogs and one very small house. These dogs weighed about 100 pounds each. The house was only about 700 square feet and was crowded with furniture.

"On rainy days, we would leave the dogs inside the house, because the yard would get so muddy, and so would they. My wife would usually come home from work earlier than I, and the house would be trashed. Once, they emptied all the stuffing out of a Lazy Boy recliner. I couldn't tell until I sat in it because they had made a nice neat pile of foam behind the chair. When my wife came home from work, and the house was trashed, she would smack them on the nose with a newspaper, and then make them sit in the bathtub for an hour as punishment. I would come home an hour later, and the dogs would be sitting in the bathtub looking to me to grant parole.

"One day she called me at work and said she couldn't find the dogs anywhere. The house was trashed, but no dogs. I said to look around the neighborhood, and if she couldn't find them I would come home and help look. She called back a few minutes later and said she had found the dogs. I asked her where they were, thinking they had been running around outside. She had found them in the bathtub. What do you make of that?"

"I have no idea," said Bob.

"Well, what do you think my wife and I were trying to teach them."

"Obviously, you didn't want them trashing the house."

"And what do you think they learned?"

"I'm not sure."

"They were pretty smart dogs. They figured that if they trashed the house and then got in the bathtub, they might not get hit with the newspaper. In this particular instance they were right. My wife and I thought it was so funny, we laughed for ten minutes on the phone."

"That's hilarious." He laughed.

"Why do you think I told you that story?"

"I'm guessing you want to make sure that I have learned the right lessons."

"Exactly."

"So tell me what you learned."

"Boy, that's a tough one. How long do you have?"

"All day."

"The most important thing I've learned is to ask myself the right questions, questions that apply to me. We spend so much time looking for answers to our lives, that we forget to examine the questions we ask. We might find answers, but they might be to the wrong questions. I think that is what you meant by success as an obstacle. I heard someone once say, 'Don't get good at something you don't want to do.' I like that. So instead of just being good at what is thrown in front of me, I want to figure out what I want to do, and then invest in myself and the people around me to make it happen. I need to find the things I want to do on a daily basis, not something I might attain in 20 years. We're not promised the next 20 years. Dave's heart problems made me realize that.

"I like it when you ask me what will I work for? That is a fundamentally different question than what's my dream, or what do I want? It keeps me grounded and helps me decide how important things are to me. It has helped me with other people as well. I need to know my staff, my family, even my bosses well enough to know what engages them. I pay attention to their behaviors to tell me about themselves. I listen when they tell me about what they want, but it is their actions that really communicate to me what's important.

"Another important thing is the notion that until I know what I want and work for it, I can't blame other people or hold them accountable for not giving me what I want. When I think back on most of my life, it makes me sad to think how I've treated some people, because they wouldn't give me what I want. The blame compromised a lot of relationships. The nice thing about knowing this now, is that my wife and my family and I are doing the work. I realize how hard it is to know what we want, especially if we haven't really experienced it. I guess that's part of the observation-statement thing you talk about. Making little observations gives me new ideas about what I want. I'm not looking to win the lottery or have some incredible dream that will change my life over night."

"What have you learned about making mistakes, about dealing with fear?"

"Let me stay with the observation piece as a way of explaining what I've learned. I make observations and have new ideas. Some of those ideas are in areas I don't really know anything about. I am successful in my job financially, and I feel some sense of competence. Having these new ideas is a little uncomfortable for me, because I know that if they are in areas of ignorance for me, I have to start out as a novice. That bothers me, because I'll have to risk being laughed at by my friends or kids. I'll have to be vulnerable, because my skill level isn't very well-developed yet."

"In those cases where does your power come from?"

"From knowing that I want to do something, that it means a lot to me, and that it is my own idea. What gets me through the most, though, is the concept of learning as engagement. Curt said something funny to me that stuck with me. He said that when little kids are in a room by themselves, they constantly try new things. They haven't had many deposits in the National Bank of Fear yet so everything is new. Failure doesn't really register as an option for them. So they try something, and they keep trying. Eventually they might even go ask for help from their parents or siblings. Failure to them is just data."

"Exactly," I jumped in. How they feel is data about what they just did, what they experienced. That's an important concept about this work. How we feel matters because it is data, our data about our lives. What we like and don't like. What is worth pursuing or working for and what's not. If you really break it down to its most simple form, the process is a way of collecting data about your life so you can make fully informed decisions."

"Why didn't you tell me that before now?" Bob wondered. He looked at me like I was holding back on him or like a puppy that tilts its head.

"Because you learned it on your own. I was just articulating it more clearly. It means more to you by discovering it than if I told you earlier."

"Well," he dove back into himself, "I try to take on new things from that perspective. If I can't do something, I learn about it and try again. I remember the lessons and forgive myself. If I have to apologize to others, I do that as well. It's easier for me to say I'm sorry, to myself and to others, if I know I will do the work to improve. I do weigh the consequences of trying something new, and if I decide it is too risky, I don't do it. The high risks are usually more external, such as injury or financial. I don't get in my own way as much, by being afraid or worrying what others think of me. I still want to treat people well. I just don't want them defining my life for me.

"I love watching people rollerblade and snowboard. My kids do both, but I always figured I was too old to learn those things. Now, I'm not saying I'll be doing half-pipes and jumps, but my kids think it's cool that I want to try. In fact I've asked them to help me learn."

"That sounds pretty vulnerable to me. They probably had you on some kind of pedestal. Must have been hard to step down off that."

"Initially it was, but the results were worth it. As long as I was on that pedestal for them, they didn't really know me. They knew their father, but they didn't know Bob. I used to think that I had a role to play with them as their father. I thought that was the only role I could play for them. But I realized that wasn't enough for them or me. I realized that I don't have any idea what they will grow up to be like. I think I'm a pretty decent man who has some successes in life. I have also made some real mistakes. It is those experiences that helped me learn. That's why your question of <u>how</u> someone knows something is as important as what they know. If all I do is tell my kids what I know, it isn't as useful. In order for them to know how I know things, they need to know more about me as a person. I think I can be that person for them, and their father at the same time."

"So you haven't wasted the last ten years of your life?"

Bob laughed. "I remember saying that to you. No not at all. It is those ten years that have allowed me to make the transition I am making now. Those ten years taught me a lot. I just never took the time to ask what I had learned, or how to use that information. I guess we all feel sorry for ourselves at one time or another, and it is easy to beat yourself up over what has happened. It's harder to celebrate the things you've done well. Not many things in life remind you of those things. I pulled out my resume the other day and looked at it. I have done a lot in my life. Usually the only time I look at my resume is when I look for another job. When you ask me 'what I'll work for,' that is probably the first thing I will do."

"And what is that exactly?"

"I'll create an environment that reminds me of the things that are right about me and the people around me. I'll create an environment that protects that. I know you can't tell me how to do that. I think that what happens, is that we start out knowing inherently something is special about each of us. That comes out when we play, when we fall in love, when we share with other people. But life is tough sometimes, and we get tired of getting beat up, as we try to become more independent. So we try to hide what's right about us to protect it. I noticed a real difference between me and the others you introduced me to."

"What's the difference?"

"When something challenges what's right about them, they fight back by being better, by making their magic stronger to confront head on the difficult time they face. What I've done is to placate the people around me, to withdraw behind some walls inside of me. I hid it away so long that I forgot what it was myself. It was difficult when you and I first started talking, because I knew I would have look inside those walls. I expected nothing to be there, no soul, no essence, no heart."

Where's The Magic?

I smiled. "I see that a lot. The real work is facing the fear that there is nothing special about us. We're afraid we will just confirm that we don't matter, that we have nothing to offer anyone else."

"I thought a lot about what you said about being adopted. When you first told me about feeling unlovable, I thought how difficult that must be, but as time passed, I realized that I felt the same way. I have just never said it out loud. I buried those feelings, and I set about trying to prove to everyone that I was lovable, that I mattered."

"How'd that work?"

"It didn't."

"Why do you think it didn't work?"

"Because the part of me that I was living in on a daily basis didn't believe it. That magic was missing. I was trying to convince everyone to love me, because I thought that was the only way I could matter to me. But you and your friends have presented me with a real paradox. If I didn't matter, if there was nothing special about me, why did I keep trying? What I think now is that the only way to matter to myself is to look at everything I've done in my life and give myself credit for having made it this far. The mere fact that I kept trying, that I felt happiness and sadness, that I could love and be loved by my wife, that I worked hard for things, tells me that I do matter to myself. Otherwise why would I have cared what others thought? Why would I have cared about anything?

"I was just looking in the wrong part of me and the rest of the world. At a fundamental level, I was doing the work. I just didn't take the time to figure out what I wanted, what I would work for. You mentioned the idea of behaviors and words. I was saying things to myself that weren't consistent with my actions. I made statements about who I was, but my behaviors didn't match my words. So I now pay more attention to my own behaviors to learn about what I really want. In fact I engage other people to help me observe myself. I take in that data and synthesize their experiences of me with my experiences. Then I ask myself, what question are my actions trying to answer?"

"Now I'm learning something."

Bob had learned a great deal and, in fact, he was teaching me something. This is one of the reasons I do what I do. Just like Curt learning from each patient about surgery, I learn a lot from the people I have interviewed and with whom I have worked. That is very fulfilling. It is also important because it evens out the playing field as far as power goes, which otherwise can get in the way of learning. They become more powerful in our relationship. We become more powerful together. "So what questions are you trying to answer now? Do you know what you will work for?"

"Kind of. You told me a story about a woman named Amy Baltzell, the woman who competed on the Mighty Mary in the America's Cup. She told you that her dream was to have a dream. I think that is where I am. I know some of the feelings I want to have: independent but connected, a sense of rhythm to my life. I remember I said to you I wanted to feel free. Part of the dream is to focus more on feeling free and exercising the freedom I have.

"I spent too much time focused on freedom *from* things. The funny part is that a lot of the things I was trying to get freedom from didn't really exist. The real obstacles were my own responses to those things. I know some things will still frighten me, but the question I now ask is how do I respond to the fear? I don't worry so much about the external event that elicited the fear. I thought of an analogy that I think you'll like."

"Let me hear it." Bob was engaged in his own process, *The Process*. His thoughts, his feelings were focused inward. He cared what I thought of his analogy, but he cared more what he thought of it. We'd come along way in a few months.

"When I was a kid, I broke my ankle, and they put a cast on it. It meant not playing hoops for a while. I really wanted to get back to playing hoops. I couldn't wait to get the cast off. Finally the day came and I attacked the rehab. Rebuilding the muscles, getting the range of motion, getting treatment. When I was done and ready to play again, the orthopedic surgeon told me how proud he was of me, of how hard I had worked rehabbing my ankle.

"When I went out to play again, I was a little scared of getting hurt, but hoops meant so much to me, it was worth the risk. A few years ago, I broke the ankle again. They put a cast on it for a while, and then I wore a walking cast. It was actually pretty comfortable. I got used to having it on. When the time came to do the rehab, I didn't want to do it, and I kept wearing the walking cast to protect it. The difference between those two experiences reminds me of how you talk about dealing with obstacles."

"How's that?"

"Well, when I was a kid, I wanted to protect my ability to play basketball, to have fun, to engage in something. I loved hoops and would do anything I could to play. I even walked a few miles a day with the cast so I could just shoot by myself. But when it happened two years ago, the only thing I cared about was avoiding the pain. I protected myself from the pain of rehab. It was easier to leave the cast on, even though the ankle was wasting away. All the muscles atrophied. I didn't notice because the cast was supporting it.

"When the doctor finally took the cast away, the rehab was ten times harder. I had avoided the initial pain, but in the long run it was worse. In the last few months I've realized how I do that to myself emotionally. When something hurts I just put a cast around what's right about me and protect it. The longer I do that, the weaker it gets. So now I want to give myself time to heal when something happens, but I need to stay in touch with what I value, that I want to share with others. I need to do the work, even if it is painful. If I don't, it will hurt more in the long run."

"Sounds pretty touchy feely to me." Bob smiled. "Can I have your permission to use that?"

"Sure. Gee, I never pictured myself as a resource for you."

"Speaking of resources, what would you say about the relationship between authorities and resources?"

"I've thought about that a lot, too. I have spent too much time giving other people authority over me. People like my boss, my family, even companies whose bills I have to pay."

"Explain that?"

"As far as other people go, I let all of them into my life because they could provide something to me. But I lose focus on that, because I haven't created the right environment to remind me of what they give me. I love my wife and family, and they love me. I spend too much time worrying about what they want from me. I've been afraid that if I don't take care of them I'll lose them. No, that's not quite right. If I don't buy them the things they want, or the house they want, or the cars they want, I'll lose them.

"Somewhere in there the love I want from them and to give them is lost. I don't experience the love, I just try to keep them around. In doing that, I just respond to what they ask for. I need to see them as a resource for the love I want, the life I want. I want them to see me that way. They probably feel the same way: that I am just an authority figure, who they have to please. There's no sense of mutuality.

"At work, it is easy to forget what a great resource my company and the people are. One day I overheard someone say how great the company was to work for. I asked her why she thought that. She said it was because the benefits are so good. I asked if she was happy there? She thought a minute and said, 'No. I guess instead of worrying about finding day care and good insurance plans, I just worry about losing them.' That hit me hard. So I went home and wrote out what I want from my company and the people I work for. You want to hear what I came up with?"

"Sure." I was learning a lot from this guy who came slinking into my office several months ago. He pulled out a daytimer.

"I can tell you talked to Curt."

"Yeah. He has a small daytimer he carries around his pocket, but not for appointments. It is for his ideas and the things he picks up from people each day. I call it my energy bank. Curt showed me his. He uses it to remember things he might forget that are important, but that he actively has to connect to. He'll go home later and work on those things. One day at work I went around and asked people what they wanted from me as their supervisor, what they had expected when they came to work for the company initially, what they hoped for everyday. I got some of the same answers you told me about. But when they saw I was being sincere, they came up with some great things. I realized that I wanted some of these same things. I narrowed my list to four categories. When I experience one of them, I write it down in this book."

Inspiration, Education, Evaluation, Compensation

"Sounds good. What are the categories?"

"Inspiration, education, evaluation, and compensation. I think they have to go in that order to work. In a sense it is the same as your process, but I have adapted it to my job."

Wow. He was giving me the advanced course on my own stuff. He had taken my ideas and applied them to his own life.

"*Inspiration* is first because without it, I could just go through the motions on all the others. I need to motivate myself, but I want my company to inspire me to use my motivation. Inspiration to me implies a bigger picture, something that touches everyone in the company. I think that is what your dad gave to his people. He took them to see those kids. He created those buttons. He included everyone as part of the team when they got licensed. I think it is important for a company to do that. I don't think they owe it to the employees, but it makes good business sense to me.

"That kind of inspiration makes people want to be better. They're connected to something bigger than they are, but what they add is themselves, so the inspiration meshes with the motivation. Too many things companies do these days challenge the motivation of the employees. I came up with that when you told me about the obstacles the medical students faced, and how you removed most of them. Being better means knowing more, acquiring new skills, and honing old ones."

"A good example from my interviews would be Bruce Hornsby," I said. "He made me think about being better. He told me a story of how when he turned forty, he reflected on where to go from there. He thought about retiring. That lasted about 10 seconds. So he said, 'What do I have to do to go to the next level?' He decided to teach his left hand to play everything his right hand could play. He sat in his studio, and showed me how difficult that was. It took him two years to do it. It was hard enough for himself, but he also had to tell his wife that he needed a few hours a day for a couple of years to be alone. He needed to practice. His wife agreed, but didn't understand. Two years went by and Bruce played a solo show in Richmond. He unveiled his new skills at that concert. His wife came backstage in tears of understanding what he had accomplished.

"The cool thing about that from my perspective, is that only a small percentage of the public could even understand or hear the new level he was at, and that his wife was one of them. I must admit I didn't really get it until I went to a show he did with Jackson Browne. They did some solo stuff and then played together. After Jackson Browne had finished playing, Bruce came out sat down and started messing around with the keys. Jackson Browne did a double take and said to the audience, 'Where did that piano come from?' Browne was surprised, because of the virtuosity of performance. I understood that night that Bruce had done this for himself and the few people who would understand it. It probably won't sell more records, but it is a true expression of who Bruce is. He did the work."

"Exactly. Being inspired makes a person want to be better. *Education* is the way to be better. You need to learn the skills and prepare. In our company, we hire great programmers, but we don't give them the tools they need to get better, to stay current with the marketplace. I want to change that. I want make sure our people have the tools and the skills, and education is the only way to do that.

"Which leads me to *Evaluation*. It seems to me that too much of the conversation at work is about how we are evaluated. That actually ties into compensation. We get evaluated and then compensated based on that evaluation. I think that inspiring and educating people gives us the right to evaluate them. I think we have that backwards too often. We think because we pay them, we have the right to evaluate them. It would be like hiring a carpenter to do job, and then saying he didn't do a good enough job, because we limited the tools he could use or the supplies or time we gave him to build the house.

"Finally, *Compensation* is not just financial. You said at the bar one day that studies show that most people who feel they aren't paid fairly will be unhappy. You also said that above a level that people feel is unfair, money is not a major factor in the levels of happiness at work, so even if companies could pay more, it wouldn't solve the problem. I want to find ways to compensate people emotionally, to tap their internal sources of motivation. In fact, I've called a staff meeting next week to discuss ways to boost morale, to engage people at work. I'd like to be able to talk with you about those things some time"

"That sounds great. It would be a pleasure." I wished I had been taping this time with him. I could feel a sense of sadness welling up through me. Time to let him go. I had picked the top of the mountain on purpose because he was ready to fly on his own. When Curt talks about teaching his residents, he calls it teaching them to fly. Bob was soaring.

Bob started to say something, but I stopped him. "I want to say thanks, Bob. You've taught me a lot. Not to sound condescending, but I'm proud of you. You've given me a lot."

"What could I have possibly given you?"

"You reminded me that an adopted kid could make a difference no matter what ghosts are flying around in his head. We talked about connecting, about making a difference, about knowing that you matter. Working with you reminds me of the lessons I have learned, and all the pain I've been through learning those things, and the compensation that brings. Working with people connects everything together, the good times, the bad times, even the feelings of being unlovable. You remind me of the parts of me I value. You allowed me to enjoy my talent because you did the work. Thanks."

"Wow. I had this speech prepared to give you, but…"

"You're welcome."

Bob and I walked off the mountain in silence. Bob paused at the bottom to take in the lake and the hawk soaring in the thermals.

"Easy Speed."

He climbed into his car and started to drive away. I could hear him singing, but couldn't quite make it out. He paused at the end of the driveway and waved goodbye. I could hear him more clearly now. "Meet George Jetson. Jane his wife," the theme song from the Jetsons.

Renewing My Lease

I walked to the street and grabbed my mail from the box. As I walked down the gravel driveway, Jazz and Righteous ran circles waiting for me to cross their invisible fence. Boo chased Raige out from the tall grass along the driveway. They paused and waited for me, as I walked along opening my mail. A nondescript envelope contained my yearly lease renewal. I thought about the financial consequences of renting versus owning. Straight out of college and even early in grad school, my wife and I had always owned houses. At one point, we owned two houses. Now I was renting an old farmhouse on four and a half acres of land in the mountains next to a lake. What were the trade-offs?

Would owning a house make more sense for me? Why do so many people talk about having a mortgage, but rarely mention their house?

The yearly commitment of signing a lease was a catalyst to make me think my life through for at least the next few years. Signing up for another year made me ask myself if I truly was where I wanted to be, doing what I wanted to do. It made me think about the next three or four years, and where I had been in my past. Reviewing the lease was a simple way to process and learn from the past, to live in the present, and to move toward the future I wanted. Watching my personal zoo follow me back to the house, running around me in circles, skirmishing with each other, I knew whatever I would do would include these guys.

People always ask, "How're you doing?" Some of them mean it for more than just words of greeting. I could honestly answer that my life was pretty simple. Maybe the Easy Speed was missing at times, but the inherent simplicity in my life allowed me to take advantage of the opportunities that came along, and that I was prepared for. I expected to have to be engaged at least once every day of my life. I expected that, because I know how to create that for myself.

The most important lesson no one ever taught me was that how I felt mattered, that it impacted every facet of my life. I had learned from some of the most successful people on the planet that how I felt mattered, that knowing how I wanted to feel was my responsibility, and that doing what it took to feel that way was not a selfish endeavor, but set me up to help others in a way that the old shut-down me never could. I learned that deciding to pursue things because of how they made me feel allowed me to identify how I wanted to feel and hold onto that "feel."

I also realized in listening to other people that much of the dissonance in our lives is the result of being told to ignore how we feel, to get tough, to hunker down. That would be great if we did not feel our lives. The reality is we do feel our lives and what I learned was not to hide from that feel, but to accept that it means something. My responsibility, the freedom I could give myself, came from paying attention, collecting data about my life, and then making informed decisions, informed in a way that included how I felt. Collect the data and put the passion to work.

I learned to differentiate between a feel that was useful and a feel based on impulsiveness that was indeed selfish and led to undesirable consequences. I accepted the fact that I do, in fact, feel and that was merely data for me to act on or not. Like the proclamation by Descartes

"I think therefore I am," and William James's claim that his first act of free will was to believe that it existed, this lesson was my personal exclamation, my Declaration of Independence. Freedom buttressed by responsibility. Achievement invigorated by expression. A Social Contract with myself. Goals given meaning by an underlying dream, a dream defined and refined by how I wanted to feel.

So many people I know and have worked with fill their lives with busy work. They do it for many reasons, but, too often, it is merely to distract themselves from the shortcomings in their lives, or their fear that they are not good enough, or from sheer boredom with their lives. In being busy, they lose their flexibility, their freedom. By living that way, they do not create their own luck. They are unprepared for the opportunities that might come their way. They may achieve some successes, but short-term successes become obstacles themselves, drawing people further away from a view of themselves they would cherish.

Sure, I'd love to be sharing my life with that special person. I'd love to be making decisions with the right woman. It would be easy to berate myself for being divorced and single at age thirty-eight. The truth for me is that I hadn't so much failed in my past relationships, as that I just wasn't prepared. I hadn't been able to give myself to someone earlier in life, because I didn't have myself to give. When Larisa came along, I was ready, but she wasn't. Perhaps we weren't right for each other no matter how ready either of us was.

Jazz tackled Righteous from behind at full speed. Boo and Raige squared off with each other, sat on their hind legs, and hissed. The work I have done thus far on myself is certainly incomplete. My standing civil war still exists, but it's essence, its purpose, are clearer for me, because I can better articulate the two sides. In his biography of T. E. Lawrence, Robert Graves describes two views of Lawrence that capture my own struggle. On one hand, he describes Lawrence this way:

People like Lawrence are an obvious menace to civilization; they are too strong to be dismissed as nothing at all, too capricious to be burdened with a position of responsibility, too sure of themselves to be browbeaten, but then too doubtful of themselves to be heroes.[13]

---

[13] Robert Graves, Lawrence and the Arabs (New York: Paragon House, 1991)

Later in his book, Graves describes Lawrence more benevolently:

The least and most that can be said about Lawrence is that he is a good man. This good is something that can be understood by a child or a savage or any simple-minded person. It is just a feeling you get from him, the feeling that here is a man with great powers, a man who could make most men do for him exactly whatever he desired, but yet one who would never use his powers, from respect for the other man's freedom.[14]

Two views of the same man, both accurate, but seemingly contradictory. Both views are part of the process: our dreams and the obstacles along the way. We are challenged to hold onto the dreams and accept the obstacles. All of us dream, all of us face obstacles. The difference between those who make it and those who don't, lies in the preparation, the work they'll do to hold onto the dream and to learn from the obstacles.

That is what I learned from the people I interviewed: life is not static; it is an ongoing activity that can be shaped to fulfill your dream. But a dream without preparation is a heavy burden; it raises doubts that we may not be good enough. Preparation without a dream is simply work. Obstacles without dreams revisited are killers. Curt, Jeff, John, and hundreds of others synthesized these seemingly contradictory aspects of life into a meaningful process in their own lives. I have translated that into an explicit process for my life and have shared it with others.

I reached into my car and pulled out a pen. I signed my name to the lease. I was where I wanted to be, doing what I wanted to do.

---

[14] Ibid.

1. T. E. Lawrence, Seven Pillars of Wisdom
2. Malcolm Gladwell, The Physical Genius (The New Yorker, August, 1999).
3. William James, Psychology: The Briefer Course (Indiana: University of Notre Dame Press, 1985).
4. Ibid.
5. Walt Whitman, Leaves of Grass (New York, The Penguin Group).
6. Jon Wild, Uncut
7. Hans-Georg Gademer, Truth and Method (New York: The Continuum Publishing Company, 1994).
8. Ibid
9. Alexis de Tocqueville, De la Democratie en Amerique (On Democracy in America) (New York: Plenum Press).
10. Jacob Needleman, Money and the Meaning of Life (New York: Doubleday Books, 1994)
11. T. E. Lawrence, Seven Pillars of Wisdom (USA: First Anchor Books, 1991).
12. Dean Ornish
13. Robert Graves, Lawrence and the Arabs (New York: Paragon House, 1991)
14. Ibid.

Made in the USA
Lexington, KY
29 March 2012